WEREWOLVES, AND DEMONS

VAMPIRES, WEREWOLVES, AND DEMONS

Twentieth Century Reports in the Psychiatric Literature

Richard Noll

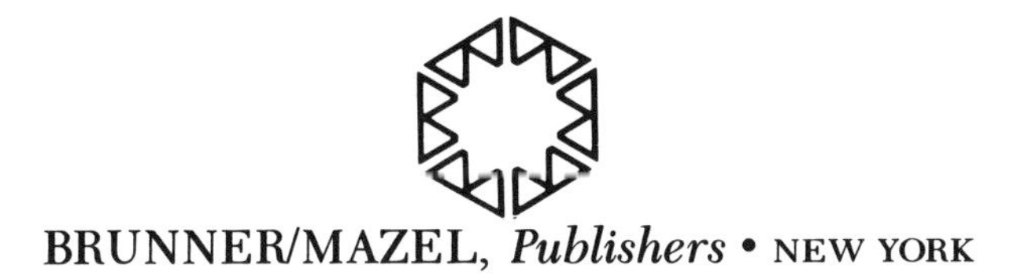

BRUNNER/MAZEL, *Publishers* • NEW YORK

Library of Congress Cataloging-in-Publication Data
Vampires, werewolves, and demons : twentieth century reports in the psychiatric literature / [edited by] Richard Noll.
p. cm.
Includes bibliographical references.
ISBN 0-87630-702-0 (pbk.)—ISBN 0-87630-632-6
1. Vampires—Case studies. 2. Werewolves—Case studies. 3. Demonomania—Case studies. 4. Vampires—Psychology. 5. Werewolves—Psychology. 6. Demoniac possession—Psychological aspects. 7. Psychiatry—Miscellanea. I. Noll, Richard.
BF1556.V36 1991
616.89—dc20 91-26933
CIP

Published by
BRUNNER/MAZEL, INC.
19 Union Square
New York, New York 10003

MANUFACTURED IN THE UNITED STATES OF AMERICA

10 9 8 7 6 5 4 3 2

For three wise men . . .
Abraham Van Helsing, M.D.
Lankester Merrin S.J.
C.G. Jung, M.D.

CONTENTS

FOREWORD

Mr. Richard Noll, M.A., a clinical psychologist, has produced the following fascinating study of three highly taboo subjects, namely, vampires, lycanthropes, and the demonically possessed. As he correctly points out, what definitely unites them is the assumption that evil is at the root of all three, and that is a key observation: The drinking of human blood, the eating of human flesh, and acting as if controlled by a devil-inside are, after all, basically dangerous, antisocial activities. The afflicted patients must be treated, even though the cure rate of such cases, as the reader will see, is apparently very low.

Having written four books on the historical sadist Vlad Dracula and a collection of the best vampire stories from history and literature over the past two thousand years, I have always had a decent fear of living vampires, cannibals, and devil-possessed humans. It is good to see that Mr. Noll shares those fears with me, and that he also agrees with Dr. Abraham van Helsing in Stoker's *Dracula* novel that "the superstitions of yesterday become the scientific truths of today" and that "we have far more in common with our healing brethren of ages past than we may like to admit."

Mr. Noll brings to his topics both an open mind and a childhood fascination with monsters. Both of these traits I hope I share with him, since I believe these traits are necessary in a search for bizarre truth. As Stephen King has young Mark Petrie say in *Salem's Lot*, "Death is when the monsters get you!" One should, I feel, have a healthy respect for monsters, both real and imaginary.

The citation of Jung's statement in his book that "clinical diagnoses are important, since they give the doctor a certain orientation . . . [but] they do not help the patient. The crucial thing is the story," should be written over doorways and broadcast on television screens to be viewed especially in medical hospitals and doctors' offices. The emphasis should be on the patient's own story, not on the technical terms of clinical diagnoses, because words, however sophisticated or scientific they may seem, generally cannot cure a patient in and of themselves. Some modern psychiatrists wrongly treat mental illness designations like magic, as if the mere pronouncement of the disease would drive the demons away.

There is still so much we do not know and do not understand about human behavior, as Mr. Noll correctly points out. It is, after all, rather significant that extensive outbreaks of the cases of vampirism rose historically not during the Dark Ages but precisely during the modern period of the Enlightenment. It often seemed as if humans were breaking under the strain of too much rationality and the weight of too many so-called "scientific" explanations.

Mr. Noll has previously done extremely important research on shamanism, following the lead of the great Mircea Eliade, who held that the oldest and most widespread of all the occult traditions is shamanism and that modern psychotherapeutic practice is often a kind of shamanism dressed up in a culturally modified form. As Noll puts it, "Telling a patient that his or her distress is due to the unseen [occult] influence of the unconscious id impulse is no different than a shaman telling a patient that his or her distress is due to the intrusion of magical disease objects . . . ."

I salute this pioneer work into the hidden deep recesses of the human mind. It is not for the squeamish. Reading this research into the gory may sometimes elicit emotions akin to the shock of splatterpunk in contemporary music. It is frightening but uncannily true.

Dr. Raymond T. McNally
Boston College
Department of History
Chestnut Hill, Mass.

ACKNOWLEDGMENTS

The purpose of this book is to remind psychiatrists and psychologists that there is still uncharted territory to explore in the shadowlands of human nature. We have far more in common with our healing brethren of ages past than we may like to admit. Biological psychiatry can shed little light on the individual case histories in this book; they are 20th century atavisms of a supernatural psychopathology that were long thought only to be the concern of folklorists, anthropologists, and historians of the occult. These stories should give us pause when we swell with pride over our remarkable ability to translate the signs and symptoms of mental disorders into biochemical and neurophysiological metaphors. I am in full agreement with William James when he admits (in an 1879 letter included in the introductory section on Demoniacal Possession in this book), "I am convinced that we stand with all these things at the threshold of a long enquiry, of which the end appears as yet to no one, least of all myself."

I have long had an interest in the horror genre, and in particular how so many of the themes that appear in its books and movies reflect important truths about the human psyche. A childhood fascination with the magazine *Famous Monsters of Filmland* has finally borne fruit in adulthood as I amplify the archetypes of the horror genre (vampires, lycanthropes, and the possessed) in the modern complaints and suffering of real people for whom vampirism, lycanthropy, and demonic possession are real afflictions.

I am indebted to William James for continually clarifying my thinking on so many matters. Before working on any psychological issue I always consult his *magnum opus*, which is now a century old.

There are many people in my life who have stimulated my thinking on the matters discussed in this book and I consider them all mentors: Leonard George, Ph.D., of Vancouver, British Columbia, is always the "bearer of light" and, although a psychologist by training, has an exemplary grasp of the historical literature on ancient and medieval European heresy and dissent as well as the psychological underpinnings of the technologies of so-called "occult" traditions. Frank W. Putnam, M.D., has encouraged me to explore unpopular hypotheses when it comes to multiple personality and the dissociative disorders, and I have valued his advice. Katherine Ramsland, Ph.D., Norman Cohn, Ph.D., Jeffrey Burton Russell, Ph.D., Andrew Samuels, Bram Stoker, William Peter Blatty, Clive Barker, Stephen King, Raymond McNally, Ph.D., Radu Florescu, Ph.D., Colin Ross, M.D., Gábor Klaniczay, Ph.D., Andrzej Wiercínski, Ph.D., and Mihály Hoppál, PhD., have all inspired me through their advice and writings.

My interest in the vampire legend also stems in part from my ancestral roots in Transylvania (Siebenbürgen) on both sides of my family. My paternal grandmother's family were German Saxons from Transylvania, and although their surname was Herman I do not know if there is a connection with the important Transylvanian city of Hermannstadt (now Sibiu in Romania). I do know that my grandmother, Sarah (Herman) Noll (1906–1990), visited our Transylvanian Saxon relatives in Romania in the mid-1960s in the village of Tirnaveni (formerly Diciosanmartin or Dicsö-Szt. Marton). The village is on the river known as the Tirnava Mica, which is a very short distance from the town of Sighisoara (Schässburg), the birthplace of the actual 15th century historical Dracula, Vlad the Impaler. Some of my distant Transylvanian ancestors may have been impaled by Dracula, a Wallachian (Romanian) prince, during the ethnic violence he led against the German Saxons between 1457 and 1460. My great-grandmother, Anna Svet, who was the mother of my maternal grandfather Stanley Adamczak (1908–1957), was a Rom (gypsy) born in Transylvania when it belonged to Hungary at the end of the last century.

I have dedicated this book to three "wise old men." Although two of them are fictional characters, they served as role models for me when I was an adolescent. I was impressed by their combination of scientific/medical expertise and their thorough knowledge of the anomalies of human nature that are generally devalued and relegated to the shadowlands as "occult" or "supernatural" topics of little scientific concern. C. G. Jung, of course, was a living human being, but alas, I have only met him through his writings and the written reminiscences of those who knew him personally. The Jung I know is only a shade, a personal construction in my imagination. Yet, his words have been profoundly influential in the development of my own thought, and in the meditations that precede and accompany my scholarly work, it is his voice that is the *aliquem alium internum* that guides my research and gives me the courage to speculate on and entertain highly unusual insights into many, many different areas of human experience.

I hope that you find something of value in this book, and I especially wish that you find as much enjoyment in reading it as I did in writing and editing it.

Haddonfield, N.J.
31 October 1990

INTRODUCTION

"There are mysteries which men can only guess at, which age by age they may solve only in part."

Abraham Van Helsing, M.D.,
in Bram Stoker's novel, *Dracula*
(Chapter 15), 1897

Just when psychiatry seems to be on the verge of exciting discoveries about the genetic, biochemical, and neurophysiological basis of so many of the mental disorders that have plagued humankind since the beginning of recorded history, it is ironic that the medical and psychiatric journals have been reporting—and with increasing frequency—baffling case histories of persons who seem to be suffering from mysterious afflictions that have been documented for thousands of years and that have long been regarded as supernatural in origin.

Vampirism, lycanthropy ("werewolfism"), and demonic possession are three such disorders attributed to occult or supernatural causes that have been reported in the past several decades in the published clinical reports of psychologists, psychiatrists, and other mental health professionals. Why it is that ancient "supernatural" afflictions are still being reported with such frequency in the "scientific" 20th century is unknown.

Perhaps the value of studying the individual case histories of persons with these unusual psychiatric syndromes lies in the fact that they tend to restore an interest in the subjective experience of mental disorders, indeed in the uniquely human characteristics of such experiences, an emphasis that late 20th century psychiatry often seems to ignore as more and more space in the professional journals is devoted to research reports involving large numbers of subjects on which some somatic hypothesis is being tested. The case histories in this book do not fit easily into the schemata of the *Diagnostic and Statistical Manual of Mental*

Disorders, Third Edition, Revised (American Psychiatric Association, 1987), although they have been reported from time to time for many centuries and are a familiar part of the folklore of our culture. Anyone who has sampled the horror genre of contemporary novels and motion pictures will be familiar with the modern fictional depictions of vampires, lycanthropes, and the possessed. However, these disorders predate mass media's exposure of these topics, and in many instances the clinical case histories of today more closely match the case reports of centuries past than modern dark fantasies of film and literature. Further, these cases sometimes cannot be easily reduced to organic mental disorders or other categories of psychiatric nomenclature. Perhaps the wise observation of Swiss psychiatrist and analytical psychologist C. G. Jung (1875–1961) should be kept in mind: "Clinical diagnoses are important, since they give the doctor a certain orientation . . . [but] they do not help the patient. The crucial thing is the story" (cited in Samuels, 1989, p. 14).

What distinguishes the three syndromes represented in this book—all long thought to be extinct—is the ancient notion that they are not only of supernatural origin, but that the extramundane forces that cause these diseases are malevolent ones. Evil—in the most primitive sense of the idea—is at the root of vampirism, lycanthropy, and demonic possession. In medieval and Renaissance Europe, it was believed that Satan or Lucifer himself was directly responsible for these curses, and that vampires, werewolves, and evil spirits were merely the earthly agents of the Devil (for exemplary scholarship of the development of the Judeo-Christian notion of personified evil, see the four-volume history of the Devil by Russell, 1977; 1981; 1984; 1986). Even today, if the self-reports of the 20th century patients described in the case histories in this book are examined, references are often made by them to such primal notions of ego-dystonic "evil" or "satanic" forces that are influencing them to act in frighteningly bizarre and painful ways. Within the civilized breast of every 20th century human, it seems, still beats the heart of a primitive. Jung puts forth a similar idea in his 1931 essay on "Archaic Man":

> . . . it is not only primitive man whose psychology is archaic. It is the psychology also of modern, civilized man, and not merely of individual "throw-backs" in modern society. On the contrary, every civilized human being, however high his con-

> scious development, is still an archaic man at the deeper levels of his psyche. Just as the human body connects us with the mammals and displays numerous vestiges of earlier evolutionary stages going back even to the reptilian age, so the human psyche is a product of evolution which, when followed back to its origins, shows countless archaic traits. (1931/1970, p. 232)

Jung, of course, is hinting here at his concept of the collective unconscious. "We have to distinguish between a personal unconscious and an *impersonal* or *transpersonal unconscious*. We speak of the latter also as the *collective unconscious*, because it is detached from anything personal and is common to all men, since its contents can be found everywhere, which is naturally not the case with personal contents" (Jung, 1917/1926/1943/1966, p. 66). From a Jungian point of view, it is entirely plausible that periodic revivals of cases of vampirism, lycanthropy, and demoniacal possession come to the attention of psychiatry. According to him, "In so far as through our unconscious we have a share in the historical collective psyche, we live naturally and unconsciously in a world of werewolves, demons, magicians, etc., for these are the things which all previous ages have vested with tremendous affectivity" (Jung, 1917/1926/1943/1966, pp. 93–94). Thus, to understand the three unusual psychiatric syndromes represented in this volume as archaic vestiges of human psychopathology, the anthropological background to our notions of mental disease must be addressed.

PRIMITIVE CONCEPTIONS OF DISEASE

Since supernatural explanations for the causes of vampirism, lycanthropy, and demonic possession were prevalent in the Old and New Worlds long before Francis Bacon's "new philosophy" finally took hold in the 1700s (and certainly by the 1800s), it is not surprising that they resemble the disease theories of nonliterate ("primitive") societies as reported in the ethnographic literature. Indeed perhaps the mere presence of these disorders today, and the occult or supernatural interpretations that their victims offer, suggests that we are witnessing a phenomenon that may be related to archaic vestiges within the human psyche and that may be more closely related to the conventional psychology of nonliterate societies than to our technologically and psychiatrically sophisticated world.

In a classic paper published in 1932, anthropologist Forest E. Clements distinguished five primary types of "primitive concepts of disease," their accompanying treatments, and the period in cultural evolutionary history when they probably first appeared. In chronological order, these are as follows:

DISEASE THEORY	ERA OF ORIGIN	THERAPY
Disease-object intrusion	Paleolithic (early)	Extraction of disease-object
Loss of soul	Paleolithic (late)	To locate, return, and restore the lost soul
Spirit intrusion	Pleistocene (late)	a. Exorcism b. Extraction of the alien entity c. Relocation of the alien entity into another living person
Breach of taboo	Unknown	Confession, propitiation
Sorcery	Unknown	Counter-magic

If viewed within the context of these primitive theories of disease, vampirism may be related to the breach of taboo (in the sense of doing something forbidden, that is, the sexual blood-fetish phenomena that these persons manifest), whereas both lycanthropy and demonic possession are often subjectively reported to be closer to spirit intrusion than to other explanations—including modern psychiatric ones. However, if speculative analogies to the known diagnostic entities of psychiatry might be made, vampirism, as a sexually related blood fetish, would probably be classified as a type of paraphilia, whereas lycanthropy and demonic possession—both of which involve major transformations of the personality into recognizable alternate entities—would most likely fall within the amorphous not-otherwise-specified category of the dissociative disorders.

THE OCCULT ROOTS OF MODERN PSYCHIATRY

We often forget that the history of the treatment of mental illness extends far back into the past from 20th century psychiatry and psychology to the magico-religious traditions of classical, medieval, and Renaissance European heritage, and even earlier to the worldwide phenomenon of shamanism in nonliterate hunting-gathering-fishing societies. According to the noted scholar and historian of religion, Mircea Eliade, "Shamanism is the most archaic and widely distributed occult tradition" (1976, p. 56), and it has passed on its occult theories and techniques in culturally modified forms to modern psychotherapeutic practice.

The Latin-derived word *occult* made its first appearance in the English language in 1545 to refer to that which was hidden or beyond the range of apprehension, understanding, or of ordinary, everyday knowledge. A modern definition by the sociologist Edward Tiryakian (1972), which corresponds to the contemporary usage of the term, describes "the occult" in part as "intentional practices, techniques, or procedures which . . . draw upon hidden or concealed forces in nature or the cosmos that cannot be measured or recognized by the instruments of modern science. . ." (p. 498). This definition covers the domain of magico-religious practices such as shamanism and the various traditions of the classically documented practices of astrology, ritual magic, and alchemy (among many others). A broader interpretation may also include all of the hypothesized instincts, complexes, drives, archetypes, dynamisms, automatisms, covert learned behaviors, repetition compulsions, and so on, that constitute the special forces of (human) nature that are examined and altered in the course of psychotherapy, but that are also largely of more mythological than scientific (meaning, rather narrowly, directly observable and quantifiable) significance. Forces invisible to the naked eye of the afflicted patient are indeed directly felt as real in some way by that individual and are altered with the assistance of the shaman or psychiatrist or psychologist in order to heal the person and to forever change the course of personal history. The material that the clinician molds and shapes with the patient is the same quintessential "stuff," primordial clay, or *prima materia*, with which the shamans and occult practitioners worked: dreams, fantasies, imagination, memories, emotions, desires, thoughts, behaviors.

The shaman's expertise as a "master of trance" and as a "master of spirits" was what enabled him to perform the two functions necessary for the survival of his society—healing and divination—both of which involve contact with unseen (occult) forces. Through the practice of mental imagery enhancement techniques, the shaman develops what is indigenously described as an "inner" or "spiritual sight," or sometimes as a second set of eyes (the 17th century alchemist Gerhard Dorn described the analogous practice in European alchemy as learning "to see with his mental eyes," the *oculis mentalibus*). The altered states of consciousness experienced by the shaman (and often induced in his patients) that allowed him to have the vivid visions necessary to perform his journeys to retrieve lost souls, "see" into patients to diagnose their (usually mental) diseases, or execute the subsequent removal of pathogenic agents through exorcism or other means of magical extraction, all have their counterparts in modern psychotherapeutic practice. Edmonston (1986) in particular has documented the transmission of one such psychotherapeutic technique—hypnotic induction—from its shamanic and ancient civilized sources, throughout the underground occult traditions of Europe, to the animal magnetism of Mesmer, and finally, to the hypnotherapy of French alienists, who first used the word psychotherapy in about 1890 to refer to this practice. The persistence of other occult practices that were part of European alchemy, ritual magic, kabbalistic rituals (see Idel, 1988), and perhaps even the heretical activities that were deemed witchcraft are continued widely today in the use of hypnosis, guided imagery, and Jung's "active imagination" in psychotherapy (Noll, 1985; 1987).

A rather direct line of descent from the occult techniques of shamanism to modern 20th century psychotherapeutic techniques can indeed be traced through the course of cultural evolutionary history. This fact has been amply demonstrated by Henri Ellenberger in his magisterial *The Discovery of the Unconscious* (1970) and is frequently mentioned in the early chapters of volumes that summarize the history of psychiatry (e.g., Zilboorg, 1941; Alexander & Selesnick, 1966; Galdston, 1967; Rosen, 1968) and those that examine the factors common to so-called primitive and modern psychotherapeutic practices (Frank, 1961; Kiev, 1964; Torrey, 1972; Edmonston, 1986).

What is generally understated in the present age, however, is that until the mid-19th century, when Wilhelm Griesinger initiated the long reign of the Germans as leaders in psychiatry by forcefully promoting a psychopathology based solely on organic factors in dysfunctional brains, theories of the etiology and treatment of mental illness still relied primarily on quasi-magical notions that were derived from ideas prominent in the occult traditions of Europe. Despite treatises written in the self-assured "scientific" style of the day, even well into the 1800s many alienists with strong religious beliefs of their own could not rule out demonic possession as the causal agent in some cases of insanity. Lunar influences are often cited in the earliest psychiatric manuals of the late 18th and early 19th centuries, and the effect of the phases of the moon on madness has continued to be periodically examined since then (see Oliver, 1943). When Philippe Pinel stated in his 1801 treatise on insanity, the classic *Traite médico-philosophique sur l'aliénation mentale, ou la manie*, that the "usual treatment" of the insane was "bleeding, bathing and purging," he was acknowledging that the most advanced treatment of his time for mental illness was still based on the ancient antiphlogistic or humoral theory of Hippocrates and Galen that was literally thousands of years old. An excess (*plethora*) of substances in the body were the cause of madness, and so, by relieving the pressure on the mind caused by these substances, mental alienation could be treated or even cured. Although bleeding the insane through venesection or leeching continued in remote asylums in the United States and Europe well into the 1800s, by mid-century most psychiatric authorities had denounced the practice as useless (Earle, 1854). Purgatives—emetics and laxatives—were administered to institutionalized mental patients until well into the 20th century in some cases, although the humoral theory was no longer cited as justification for this treatment (see the various entries for the somatic treatments of psychotic disorders in Noll, 1991). Thus, "spirit intrusion" or "disease object intrusion" that could be alleviated by exorcism or by other means of extraction or expulsion formed the primitive basis of psychiatric practice until well into the 20th century.

Have we really advanced to the point where no occult or magical ideas underlie our modern psychiatric theories and techniques? Probably not. For whenever there is an "unknown quantity," it is human nature to fill in the gaps in understanding by projecting ideas that may reveal more about our unconscious assumptions or about the human psyche itself than about the quantifiable reality of a phenomenon. Often, theoretical constructs are anthropomorphized as their creators endow themselves with divine powers and breathe life into their intellectual progeny. For example, Sigmund Freud proposed (in his final metapsychology) that the human mind was split into at least three autonomous parts with different agendas—the ego, id, and superego—and that in our mental anguish we directly experience the vicissitudes of their autonomous activities as they clash. Nothing can distinguish the essential phenomenology of what Freud was describing from the reports of warring "spirits" or "gods" influencing the lives of the ancients, for his terms for these agents merely reflects the conventions of the culture in which he lived. "Spirits" was not an acceptable word for a causal explanation of human behavior or experience in Freud's time, and it is not an acceptable one in professional circles today. Perhaps the phenomena remain the same, but the names have been changed in translation from one culture or era to another. As C. G. Jung observes about our century, "The gods have become diseases" (1929/1968, p. 37). Or, as James Hillman (1979) succinctly points out:

> Mythology is a psychology of antiquity. Psychology is a mythology of modernity. The ancients had no psychology, properly speaking, but they had myths, the speculative tellings about humans in relation with more-than-human forces and image. We moderns have no mythology, properly speaking, but we have psychological systems, the speculative theories about humans in relation with more-than-human forces and images, today called fields, instincts, drives, complexes. (pp. 23–24)

Yet, despite a 20th century humanistic education and constant immersion in a mass media that frequently reports the latest scientific "facts" in medicine and psychiatry and their organic essence, many of the nonprofessional persons who make up clinical caseloads today plainly speak of spirits or other malevolent influences on their behaviors. "Initiated" professionals assume this is because their patients are simply ignorant of the "true" causes of their behavior described best by the special magical language of the healing specialists of our culture. The magical language of psychiatry is comprised of a vocabulary that is psychoanalytic, biochemical, neurological, psychological, genetic—yet all of these words refer to "things," things that seem to have a life of their own to the patient, but that cannot be held in the patient's hand or photographed by any machine, let alone observed directly or extracted surgically. Telling a patient that his or her distress is due to the unseen (occult) influence of an unconscious id impulse, a complex, an archetype, an automatic maladaptive behavior learned from the modeling behaviors of disordered parents, the phenotypic expression of his or her genotype, dysfunctional family interaction patterns that the person repeats without awareness, or other such theoretical constructs created to identify the nature of the motivating factors in psychopathology, is no different than a shaman telling a patient that his or her distress is due to the intrusion of magical disease objects, or of spirits, or the breaching of a familial or cultural taboo, or of the loss of a soul that must be returned to the person in the course of treatment.

As our language for explaining the nature of the pathogenic agents experienced in the phenomenal worlds of our patients remains essentially primal and somewhat occult in nature, so too do descriptions of some rare and unusual mental disorders that centuries of observation and speculation still have not satisfactorily explained.

PSYCHIATRY'S TROPICAL DISEASES: UNUSUAL PSYCHIATRIC SYNDROMES

Psychiatry has roots that are historically occult and must continue to operate within the realm of human experience that is the unexplained, the unknown, the unseen. The extraordinary phenomena to be found in the shadowlands of psychiatry sometimes do not provide a good fit with existing scientific theories or terminology. The richness of human experience is difficult to taxonomize, and therefore, the map of the known psychopathological universe is continually changing. The three syndromes presented in this volume are representative of the entities found along the blurred perimeter of the psychiatric cosmos that have been referred to as "uncommon psychiatric syndromes" (Enoch & Trethowan, 1979) or "extraordinary disorders of human behavior" (Friedmann & Faguet, 1982). These are the "tropical diseases" of psychiatry that most clinicians will never encounter even once in their lifetimes.

The three disorders selected for this volume share the distinction of being unusual psychiatric syndromes of presumed malevolent supernatural origin that were reported by the ancients but that were thought to have vanished centuries ago. The 20th century case histories included here demonstrate that this is clearly not the case, and that we cannot presume to be able to explain everything. As the fictional Prof.

Dr. Abraham Van Helsing observed when outlining the rationale for his diagnosis of vampirism to the survivors of Dracula's victims, there are indeed mysteries that age by age may only be solved in part.

REFERENCES

Alexander, F. G., & Selesnick, S. T. (1966). *The History of Psychiatry.* New York: Harper & Row.

American Psychiatric Association. (1987). *Diagnostic and Statistical Manual of Mental Disorders. Third Edition, Revised* Washington, D.C.: American Psychiatric Association.

Clements, F. E. Primitive concepts of disease. (1932). *University of California Publications in American Archaeology and Ethnology, 32,* 185–252.

Earle, P. Bloodletting in mental disorder. (1854). *American Journal of Insanity, 10,* 387–405.

Edmonston, W. E. (1986). *The Induction of Hypnosis.* New York: John Wiley & Sons.

Eliade, M. (1976). The occult and the modern world. In Eliade, M., *Occultism, Witchcraft, and Cultural Fashions: Essays in Comparative Religions.* Chicago: University of Chicago Press.

Ellenberger, H. (1970). *The Discovery of the Unconscious.* New York: Basic Books.

Enoch, M. D., & Trethowan, W. H. (1979). *Uncommon Psychiatric Syndromes.* 2nd ed. Bristol, UK: John Wright & Sons Ltd.

Frank, J. D. (1961). *Persuasion and Healing: A Comparative Study of Psychotherapy.* Baltimore: Johns Hopkins Press.

Friedmann, C. T. H., & Faguet, R. A. (1982). *Extraordinary Disorders of Human Behavior.* New York: Plenum Press.

Galdston, I. (1967). *Historic Derivations of Modern Psychiatry.* New York: McGraw-Hill.

Hillman, J. (1979). *The Dream and the Underworld.* New York: Harper & Row.

Idel, M. (1988). *Kabbala: New Perspectives.* New Haven: Yale University Press.

Jung, C. G. (1917/1926/1943/1966). On the psychology of the unconscious. In Jung, C. G. *Two Essays on Analytical Psychology. The Collected Works of C. G. Jung, Vol. 7.* 2nd ed. Princeton: Princeton University Press.

Jung, C. G. (1929/1968). Commentary on "The Secret of the Golden Flower." In Jung, C. G., *Alchemical Studies. The Collected Works of C. G. Jung, Vol. 13.* 2nd ed. Princeton: Princeton University Press.

Jung, C. G. (1931/1970). Archaic man. In Jung, C. G., *Civilization in Transition. The Collected Works of C. G. Jung, Vol. 10.* 2nd ed. Princeton: Princeton University Press.

Kiev, A. (ed.). (1964). *Magic, Faith, and Healing: Studies in Primitive Psychiatry Today.* New York: The Free Press.

Noll, R. (1985). Mental imagery cultivation as a cultural phenomenon: The role of visions in shamanism. *Current Anthropology, 26,* 443–461.

Noll, R. (1987). Mental imagery cultivation and individuation: The historical context of techniques of spiritual transformation. In Heinze, R. I. (ed.), *Proceedings of the Third International Conference on the Study of Shamanism.* Berkeley: Independent Scholars of Asia.

Noll, R. (1991). *The Encyclopedia of Schizophrenia and the Psychotic Disorders.* New York: Facts-On-File, Inc.

Oliver, J. F. (1943). Moonlight and nervous disorders: An historical study. *American Journal of Psychiatry, 99,* 579–584.

Rosen, G. (1968). *Madness in Society: Chapters in the Historical Sociology of Mental Illness.* Chicago: University of Chicago Press.

Russell, J. B. (1977). *The Devil: Perceptions of Evil from Antiquity to Primitive Christianity.* Ithaca: Cornell University Press.

Russell, J. B. (1981). *Satan: The Early Christian Tradition.* Ithaca: Cornell University Press.

Russell, J. B. (1984). *Lucifer: The Devil in the Middle Ages.* Ithaca: Cornell University Press.

Russell, J. B. (1986). *Mephistopheles: The Devil in the Modern World.* Ithaca: Cornell University Press.

Samuels, A. (1989). *Psychopathology: Contemporary Jungian Perspectives.* London: Karnac Books.

Tiryakian, E. A. (1972). Toward the sociology of esoteric culture. *American Journal of Sociology, 78,* 491–512.

Torrey, E. F. (1972). *The Mind Game: Witchdoctors and Psychiatrists.* New York: Emerson Hall.

Zilboorg, G. (1941). *A History of Medical Psychology.* New York: W. W. Norton.

"Teach thy tongue to say,
'I do not know.'"

Moses Maimonides,
12th century A.D.

PART I

VAMPIRISM

Prof. Dr. Van Helsing: "Well, I shall tell you. My thesis is this: I want you to believe."
Dr. Seward: "To believe what?"
Prof. Dr. Van Helsing: "To believe in things that you cannot."

Bram Stoker,
Dracula (Chapter 14), 1897

Introduction

"There are such beings as vampires; some of us have evidence that they exist."

Abraham Van Helsing, M.D.,
in Bram Stoker's *Dracula*
(Chapter 18), 1897

BLOOD, RITUAL, AND A DANGEROUS FANTASY

The drinking of blood—particularly human blood—is one of the oldest taboos of the Judeo-Christian tradition. Perhaps the earliest scriptural prohibition comes from Pentateuch's book of Deuteronomy (12:23) in which specific procedures are outlined for the disposal of sacrificial animals: "Only take care not to consume the blood, for the blood is the life, and you must not consume the life with the flesh." The significance of blood as a symbol of life was used by Jesus in the New Testament accounts of the Last Supper. In the Gospel According to St. Matthew (26:26–29), the ritual that Jesus performs for the first time with his disciples invokes the powerful symbolism of blood as a life-force and, as some scholars have suggested, he may have deliberately employed the metaphor of a taboo activity as a device to further bond the group together through mutual participation in a forbidden practice. Doing so symbolizes a break with the old traditions, thus transforming the event into an initiation ritual: "'Take it and eat, This is my body.' Then he took a cup, and when he returned thanks he gave it to them. 'Drink all of you from this,' he said, 'for this is my blood.'"

Although the Christian Mass involved a ritualized reenactment of the Last Supper, the transformation of wine into blood that was then consumed by the priests and those persons attending the Mass was largely considered symbolic until the year 1215. At that time, Pope Innocent III held the Fourth Lateran Council at which it was decided that the priest participated in a genuine miracle at each Mass, for as the Council defined the new dogma: "The body and blood of Jesus Christ are truly contained under the appearance of bread and wine in the sacrament of the altar, the bread being transubstantiated into the body and the wine into the blood" (cited in Tannahill, 1975, p. 56). However, this controversial decision came back to haunt the Church as an important catalyst that helped ignite the 16th century Reformation, with Martin Luther and other Protestants believing that the symbolic nature of Jesus' words should be retained (consubstantiation).

Although there are many purported examples of the ritualized drinking of human blood and cannibalism in ethnographic and historical accounts (Hogg, 1958; James, 1933; Tannahill, 1975), the actual practice of such activities has been considered particularly execrable in Western culture. In fact, despite Western ethnocentric notions to the contrary, cannibalism enacted outside of a ritual context has been considered an anathema in almost all cultures. Furthermore, according to one scholar (Arens, 1979), anthropologists have been notoriously lax in verifying reports of cannibalism in exotic cultures, relying primarily on legends and second-hand reports rather than first-hand knowledge (or participant-observation!). A collection of essays on "the ethnography of cannibalism" edited by Brown and Tuzin (1983) also supports this more critical modern view of the phenomenon.

In fact, in Western culture, such activities have often been imagined by societal majorities to be practiced by minority subgroups—real or imaginary—that have beliefs or customs that conflict with those of the dominant majority, and this dangerous "fantasy" has contributed to mass executions, persecutions, pogroms, and witch-hunts involving the deaths of millions. British medieval historian Normal Cohn has identified the core complex of ideas that makes up this "fantasy" and has documented how, since at least the second century A.D., accusations of infantile cannibalism; the physical and sexual abuse of children; sex orgies involving adults, children, and sometimes animals; and blood-drinking rituals have been aimed at minority groups all too often in the course of European history. In the second century A.D., Christians were accused of indulging in this core group of abominations by the Romans.

Subsequently, Christians used these same tactics against the Jews (Strack, 1909; Trachtenberg, 1943; Hsia, 1988) and other groups deemed heretical for their deviant beliefs.

Cohn (1975, p. xi) described this "fantasy" thus: "The essence of the fantasy was that there existed, somewhere in the midst of the great society, another society, small and clandestine, which not only threatened the existence of the great society but was also addicted to practices which were felt to be wholly abominable, in the literal sense of anti-human." Cohn's scholarly focus has always been on the documentation of the influence of actual groups, cults, or sects that maintained beliefs and practices that either completely or partially conflicted with Church dogma and thus Christian ecclesiastical authority (Cohn, 1970; 1975). However, this fantasy has also been held by the majority about *imagined* minority groups.

As the legendary creature of supernatural origin known as the vampire (from the Hungarian, *vámpir*) has long been associated with blood drinking and other abominable practices, it is not surprising that the widespread folklore telling of a society of vampires that threatens humanity led to many documented mass hysterical vampire scares in various towns and cities in Central Europe during the 17th and 18th centuries (Klaniczay, 1987). In Hungary, the panics related to vampires eclipsed concerns about hunting witches, and so in 1766, a commission set up by Empress Maria Theresa drew up a new law forbidding any kind of witch-hunting, and in 1768, new laws forbade prosecution for any sort of magical activity. But as the well-known Hungarian scholar Gábor Klaniczay (1990) observes, "The Empress, it is worth noting, was roused to action not by the persistence or re-emergence of witch-hunting in Hungary, but by the popular panic about a new kind of monstrous being, the vampire, whose frequent appearances in neighboring Moravia had also aroused considerable interest in Vienna" (p. 170).

In his exemplary essay on the cannibalism issue, British ethnologist I. M. Lewis makes related observations about the reports of cannibalism and blood drinking from around the world when he argues, "In fact, the application of the derogatory label 'man-eater' is one of the most widely distributed methods by which the members of one group or community dissociate and distance themselves from outsiders beyond the pale" (Lewis, 1986, pp. 63–64). In Africa, where Lewis did his fieldwork in the 1950s, he found that victims of oppression would sometimes hurl these accusations against their societal superiors, particularly the white Europeans. Like the vampire panics that occurred from time to time in Europe, Africa too had its vampire scares:

> I discovered . . . the assumption, widely prevalent at that time, that many Europeans were vampire-men who sucked the blood and ate the flesh of innocent Africans. Similar concepts about cannibalistic Europeans flourished with varying degrees of intensity in east Africa . . . , southern Africa, and in the Congo, where during the Belgian period in Leopoldville the white vampire was known as the 'man with the lamp.' Around the same time (1958) an unsuspecting European firm in the Belgian Congo marketed canned meat in cans depicting chubby, smiling African babies. The product was not an unqualified success. (Lewis, 1986, pp. 64–65)

An excellent summary of the approach of the British social anthropologists to the issue of witchcraft accusations in Europe and in nonliterate societies is contained in the volume of essays edited by Mary Douglas (1970).

As an aside, it must be mentioned that an analogous mass hysterical phenomenon peculiar, it seems, to the United States and Canada is the frightening—but totally unsubstantiated—belief that there is a vast underground conspiracy of satanic cults practicing the Black Mass with ritualized cannibalism, the killing and eating of infants, sexual orgies involving all ages and species, and blood rituals. Reports began to appear with alarming frequency in the American media after about 1980. Some anti-satanism groups have claimed that as many as 50,000 children are kidnapped, abused, and sometimes killed each year. Day-care center staff members are accused not only of sexual abuse but also of satanism, and libraries around the country are pressured by anti-satanism groups to remove books from their shelves—often children's books, especially those, for some reason, of best-selling author Shel Silverstein. Entire families involving several generations, and perhaps even entire towns, are believed by many to be secretly part of this vast underground satanic network. Some professional refereed psychiatry journals have published articles that have added to the hysteria, passing along such unsubstantiated claims that the heretical Christian groups now known as the Gnostics practiced a form of the Black Mass in the first few centuries A.D. (Hill & Goodwin, 1989). Other articles authoritatively discuss the existence of "highly structured and rigidly secretive cults" implicated in "allegiance to or worship of Satan," including, among others, "families (including multigenerational involvement)" without providing documentation for the existence of even *one* such family or even challenging the assumption that such groups exist in any critical way (e.g., Van Benschoten, 1990).

Not surprisingly, serious investigators—for example, analysts at the Federal Bureau of Investigation (Lanning, 1989;1991)—have examined the reports and have found absolutely no corroborating physical or other evidence to back up claims of an ancient underground network of satanists involved in ritualized murder, blood drinking, and child abuse. Indeed, even Jeffrey Burton Russell, a medievalist and one of the leading historians of European witchcraft, Satan, and satanism writes, "I doubt that even today widespread organization of Satanism exists, and I can assure your readers categorically that it never existed before the beginning of this century" (Russell, personal communication, 1990). This mass psychological phenomenon is now being studied by sociologists (Victor, 1989; 1990), law enforcement analysts (Hicks, 1991), folklorists (Stevens, 1989), and psychiatrists and psychologists (Gannaway, 1989; Noll, 1989; in press) in order to understand the persistence of these beliefs in the face of an overwhelming absence of corroborating evidence. Public and professional resistance to the idea that the current satanism scare may be nothing more than a modern revival of Cohn's "fantasy" is quite strong, but it must also be pointed out that even at the turn of the century Christian theologians and Papal authorities published refutations of the idea that Jews kidnapped Christian infants and used them in blood sacrifice rituals (see Lipschiltz, 1882; Roth, 1934) because many still believed it to be true. At least the Jews could be demonstrated to physically exist; satanists seem to be the vampires of 20th century America.

VAMPIRES—THE LEGEND

> "In all the darkest pages of the malign supernatural there is no more terrible tradition than that of the Vampire, a pariah even among demons. Foul are his ravages; gruesome and seemingly barbaric are the ancient and approved methods by which folk must rid themselves of this hideous pest."
>
> Montague Summers,
> *The Vampire: His Kith and Kin*, 1928

The best source of scholarly information relating to the cross-cultural study of folklore concerning the vampire or other blood-sucking demons remains the controversial work of Montague Summers (1928; 1929). Belief in malevolent supernatural entities that fed on the blood of the living seems to have been a part of the mythologies of most cultures in one form or another, and no one has matched Summers' compilation of sources. The problem, however, lies in Summers' own personal beliefs about vampires (and werewolves, witches, demons, etc.), which he interjects liberally into his texts—namely, that these supernatural entities truly exist and are agents of the Devil sent here to earth to torment humankind. Summers (reputed to be an ordained priest in the Church of England) fancied himself a modern Inquisitor of sorts, and so some of his translations from obscure texts probably should be taken with a grain of salt until a future specialist can replicate his work. As it stands now, Summers, who lived from 1880 to 1948, can still hide behind a wall of erudition.

Two relatively recent explorations of the vampire legend from scholars of folklore can be found in the works by Barber (1988) and Dresser (1989).

The first reference in the English language to vampires appears in a 1734 book called *Travels with Three English Gentlemen.* However, the definition the author uses seems to be closely based on a German text published just the year before, in Halle, by John Heinrich Zopfius. In his *Dissertatio de Vampiris Serviensibus* of 1733, Zopfius writes:

> Vampires issue forth from their graves in the night, attack people sleeping quietly in their beds, suck out all their blood from their bodies and destroy them. They beset men, women, and children alike, sparing neither age nor sex. Those who are under the fatal malignity of their influence complain of suffocation and a total deficiency of spirits, after which they soon expire. Some who, when at the point of death, have been asked if they can tell what is causing their decrease, reply that such and such persons, lately dead, have arisen from the tomb to torment and torture them. (cited in Summers, 1928, pp. 1–2)

This early description provides all the essential characteristics of the vampire legend as we still know it today.

DRACULA

Throughout the latter half of the 18th and the entire 19th centuries, vampires were the subject of many poems, stage plays, novels, and "penny dreadfuls" throughout Europe, but particularly in England (see Carter, 1975; also Summers, 1928, pp. 271–340 as it is an exemplary scholarly treatment of "The Vampire in Literature;" for the German literature see Hock, 1901). This interest was directly due to the peaking of the "vampire epidemic" in Central Europe in the 1730s (Klaniczay, 1987). Yet none of these fictional accounts surpasses the continuing influence of the most terrifying (and titillating) vampire novel of all time, *Dracula* (1897), by Irish author Bram Stoker (1847–1912).

Stoker was a prolific writer of books and short stories, but his main occupations were as the agent for Henry Irving, one of the most famous actors in the world during the late 19th century, and as business manager for London's Lyceum Theatre (see the biographies by Ludlam, 1962, and Roth, 1982). His occupation as Irving's agent required frequent travel as the star appeared in productions throughout Europe and the United States.

It was during these many travels, specifically between the years 1890 and 1896, that Stoker began to keep working notes on the characters and plot lines for a vampire novel that would later become *Dracula*, which he finished writing about a year prior to its being published in May of 1897. Stoker used the British Museum in London and various libraries as he travelled to conduct meticulous research into the legend of the vampire, the geography and customs of Transylvania (then in Hungary), and the many other details (nautical weather schedules, etc.) that would flesh out the skeleton of the novel. His working notes were sketched out on numerous slips of paper and sheets of hotel stationary. A collection of nonfiction essays on vampirism that were apparently consulted by Stoker when researching his book have been reprinted in a collection edited by Leatherdale (1987). Although it is debated whether an actual original manuscript of Stoker's *Dracula* exists (one source told me that a private collector in California owns it), some of Stoker's original notes and library research materials were discovered by the noted Dracula scholars Raymond McNally and Radu Florescu of Boston College in the 1970s in their present location—the Philip H. and A. S. W. Rosenbach Foundation on Delancy Street in Philadelphia. A summary of the character of these private and unpublished materials can be found in a recent book by these scholars (Florescu & McNally, 1989, pp. 221–234).

Transylvania is an actual place, not merely a legend. It is an area of Central Europe that was settled primarily by German Saxons centuries ago (in addition to the Hungarians, Szekelers, Romanians, and Romani or "Gypsies" that were already there), and since most of the population was concentrated in seven towns with German names it was long known as Siebenbürgen (in German, the seven cities). The classic catalog of Transylvanian coins by Adolph Resch (1901) illustrates that the Transylvanian coat of arms of seven circles or seven fortress towers appeared on the obverse of coins depicting various Hapsburg monarchs. These were the type of coins in use in this domain of the Holy Roman Empire (*sacrum romanum imperium*) during the time of the vampire scares of the 17th and particularly the 18th centuries. Stoker uses the German names of the Transylvanian towns that were still in the Austro-Hungarian Empire of his day. However, after WWI, Transylvania was taken from Hungary and made a part of Romania and the original names of the towns were replaced by Romanian names.

McNally and Florescu are perhaps the two most important scholars ever in the study of Dracula and the vampire legend, for they also proved conclusively that Stoker's book and main character were based on actual places and people. In a 1972 book, *In Search of Dracula*, they proved that a 15th century prince of Wallachia (now a part of Romania) named Vlad Tepes (1431–1476), or Vlad the Impaler, was actually called Dracula or a variant thereof during his lifetime. "Dracul" means "dragon" or "devil," and so "Dracula" means "son of the dragon" or "son of the devil." McNally and Florescu were able to demonstrate that Stoker was aware of this real Dracula and that he based the physical description of his fictional "king of the vampires" on this 15th century prince noted and feared for impaling his enemies on wooden stakes. These two gifted scholars have contributed many classic books on the real and fictional Draculas (McNally & Florescu, 1972; Florescu & McNally, 1973; McNally, 1983; Florescu & McNally, 1989).

Stoker's *Dracula* is an extremely important work for two connections it makes that are essential to the understanding of the case histories of the clinical vampires of today: (1) the linkage of psychiatry and folklore, that is, "insanity" and vampirism; and (2) the fusion of sexual excitement and the drinking of blood.

A fact that is not frequently elaborated upon in the scholarship on

Dracula is that the nexus for the development of many events in the book is an asylum for the insane in England, and several of the characters in the book have an intimate connection with this "mad-house" (actually a large private lunatic asylum in Purfleet) whether as a patient (R. M. Renfield) or as medical professionals who live in or near its grounds (the young superintendent of the asylum, John Seward, M.D.) and their friends and loved ones (the female victims of Dracula).

In reviewing Stoker's personal papers for *Dracula* at the Rosenbach Foundation (as I did in October 1990, with my gratitude expressed to Rosenbach archivist Leslie Morris), it became immediately clear that Stoker meant his novel to have this peculiar psychiatric basis, and it was apparent from the start that the characters of an asylum physician and a psychotic patient would figure prominently. It is obvious from Stoker's notes where he got his geographical and cultural materials, but no psychiatric texts are mentioned as having been consulted even though he uses the psychiatric terminology of his day correctly and his descriptions of the psychotic Renfield's blood drinking accurately match the case histories of clinical vampirism found in the psychiatric literature (and which are included in this volume).

The assertion by Florescu and McNally (1989) that Stoker's notes at the Rosenbach Foundation contain "a few remarks about the sketches of the symptoms of insanity garnished from one of Stoker's brothers, Sir William Thornley, a former president of the Royal College of Surgeons" (p. 222) is not correct. The notes to which they refer are neurological, not psychiatric, and concern the sequelae of head trauma to various parts of the brain (e.g., contralateral symptoms, coma) and do not contain any hint of reference to the signs or symptoms of the recognized mental disorders of the late 19th century. Extensive quotations from a two-volume book on *The Theory of Dreams* (1808) by F. C. and J. Rivington is the only reference in Stoker's notes that is remotely psychological in nature, and the quotes that he reproduced from that source tend to be rather metaphysical and not very psychological. The publication of Stoker's notes in book form is presently the goal of Dracula scholar Joseph Bierman.

In the novel *Dracula*, whose plot is revealed in a series of excerpts from diaries and letters, the opening sequence takes place in Transylvania where Jonathan Harker meets the vampires for the first time in the castle of Count Dracula, but much of the action begins after Dracula buys the abandoned Carfax estate next to the asylum and courts the psychotic Renfield, who escapes his "straight-waistcoat" and his padded room repeatedly, sometimes ending up in the abandoned estate now belonging to Dracula. After Dracula's relocation to Carfax (unknown, of course, to the main characters), the fiancée of a friend of John Seward's, Lucy Westerna, develops a strange illness that causes her to sleepwalk and renders her rather anemic. She is obviously being drained of blood bit by bit during the nocturnal visits of her demon lover—Dracula. Seward, a physician, cannot find anything wrong with her, and so, as he writes in a letter, "I have written to my old friend and master, Professor Van Helsing, of Amsterdam, who knows as much about obscure diseases as anyone in the world" (Chapter 9). Van Helsing, besides being a medical expert and a professor, is an expert on the occult and he makes the supernatural diagnosis of *vampirism* and begins to treat Lucy accordingly, but without letting the others know the true cause of her distress until much later.

It is through Dracula's telepathic influence on the weak mind of the mentally ill Renfield that Dracula is able to gain entry into the asylum and into the lives of those connected with it. This aspect of the story is consistent with the theory found in Johann Wier's *De Praestigiis Daemonum (On the Wiles of the Devil)* of 1563 that the devil (and vampires are agents of the devil) usually chooses as his victims those suffering from melancholic or hysterical delusions, rendering them vulnerable to infernal deception (see Anglo, 1976). According to Stoker's reading of the vampire legend, vampires must be "invited" into a house by someone who lives there. However, prior to Dracula's arrival in England (which he plans to "conquer" and transform its inhabitants into a society of vampires), Renfield was already well on his way to becoming a clinical vampire, and in the figure of Renfield, Stoker provides a human counterpart to the supernatural vampire, the centuries-old Dracula. As they are of like natures, it was only to be expected that they would be drawn to one another, at least telepathically. Renfield, age 59, is first described in the book by Dr. Seward as having the following symptoms: "Sanguine temperament; great physical strength; morbidly excitable; periods of gloom ending in some fixed idea which I cannot make out." Stoker here reveals his informed knowledge of 19th century psychiatric nomenclature by expertly describing the classic symptoms (in Renfield) of "monomania," the most frequently diagnosed mental disorder in Europe until "hysteria" came into vogue in the last quarter of that century (see Goldstein, 1987). The monomaniacal "fixed idea" that Seward later discovers is Renfield's mad theory of perpetual life, that by ingesting the life-force of other living things his own life-force can be increased. Renfield starts by attracting flies with sugar, eating some of them himself but also feeding them to spiders, which he systematically fattens up and eats. He keeps careful calculations of the total number of lives he has consumed in a notebook, which is described to be like an accounting ledger. However, eventually the blood of flies and spiders is not enough. He asks Seward for a kitten or a cat, and is refused. Undaunted, Renfield figures out a way to attract birds to the window of his cell, but one day they disappear, although their feathers are all over his cell. Seward chillingly writes in his diary:

> 11 a.m.—The attendant has just been to me to say that Renfield has been very sick and has disgorged a whole lot of feathers. "My belief is, doctor," he said, "that he has eaten his birds, and that he just took and ate them raw!"

Although only Van Helsing can make the supernatural diagnosis of vampirism in the case of Dracula and his victims (Lucy, Mina, etc.), and Seward must invent a new psychiatric diagnosis for his human patient, the motivation of their abnormal behaviors is the same—the ingestion of the life-force (blood) of living beings to sustain their own lives. With these two vampiristic characters—one human, one supernatural—Stoker successfully weds psychiatry and folklore, clinical and legendary phenomena, and yet is true to the unique image of vampires drawn by each of these traditions.

After Renfield eats living birds, Seward excitedly writes in his diary that his "homicidal maniac is of a peculiar kind," and that he "shall have to invent a new classification for him, and call him a zoöphagous (life-eating) maniac; what he desires is to absorb as many lives as he can" (Chapter 6). Seward then becomes a bit grandiose himself, speculating that if he could unlock the secret of the mind "of even one lunatic," he could surpass the scientific achievement of "Burdon-Sanderson's physiology or Ferrier's brain knowledge." It is not known if Stoker's brother provided him with these nonpsychiatric references, although David Ferrier's *The Functions of the Brain* of 1886 was much discussed just prior to the period that Stoker began writing, as it is a clinical and experimental review of findings in support of the much-debated idea of the localization of function in the brain.

Finally, Renfield no longer remains content with ingesting insects and smaller mammals and instead succumbs to his first true act of clinical vampirism, with Seward as his victim. Seward writes in his diary:

> I was engaged after dinner in my study posting up my books, which, through press of other work and the many visits to Lucy, had fallen sadly into arrear. Suddenly the door was burst open, and in rushed my patient, with his face distorted with passion. I was thunderstruck, for such a thing as a patient getting of his own accord into the Superintendent's study is almost unknown. Without an instant's pause he made straight at me. He had a dinner-knife in his hand, and, as I saw he was dangerous, I tried to keep the table between us. He was too quick and too strong for me, however; for before I could get my balance he had struck at me and had cut my left wrist rather severely. Before he could strike again, however, I got in my right and he was sprawling on his back on the floor. My wrist bled freely, and quite a little pool trickled on the carpet. I saw that my friend was not intent on further effort, and occupied myself binding up my wrist, keeping a wary eye on the prostrate figure all the time. When the attendants rushed in, and we turned our attention to him, his employment positively sickened me. He was lying on his belly on the floor licking up, like a dog, the blood which had fallen from my wounded wrist. He was easily secured, and, to my surprise, went with the attendants quite placidly, simply repeating over and over again: "The blood is the life! The blood is the life!" (chapter 11).

Renfield's macabre theory that the ingestion of "life" (blood) is necessary for sustaining his own is repeated by some clinical vampires in their published case histories, as is zoophagous activity (e.g., drinking the blood of animals from an abattoir), which sometimes seems to precede the graduation to desiring human blood. Even though nothing is known about Renfield's childhood or history prior to being placed in an asylum, it is interesting that Stoker's character manifests the graduation of presenting symptomatology of clinical vampirism in adults as we know it today (see especially the three case histories presented by

South African psychiatrists Hemphill and Zabow reproduced in this section).

Stoker makes a second major contribution to understanding the psychology of the vampire by graphically illustrating the sexual component of drinking blood. As is discussed in the following, and in the case histories, clinical vampirism often involves a combination of sexual activity and blood drinking, and the act of drinking blood is sexually arousing, making clinical vampirism a sort of sexual blood fetish.

In *Dracula*, scenes in which a vampire seizes and bites his or her victim are described by Stoker with a boldly erotic style that seems to depict passionate acts of oral sex. Jonathan Harker gets it from one of three lovely female vampires in Dracula's castle who playfully argue over who gets to "kiss" the young man first early in the book (Chapter 3). Harker did not know they were vampires and was no doubt expecting quite another experience than the one he received:

> I lay quiet, looking out under my eyelashes in an agony of delightful anticipation. The fair girl advanced and bent over me till I could feel the movement of her breath upon me. . . . I was afraid to raise my eyelids, but looked out and saw perfectly under the lashes. The girl went on her knees, and bent over me, simply gloating. There was a deliberate voluptuousness which was both thrilling and repulsive, and as she arched her neck she actually licked her lips like an animal, till I could see in the moonlight the moisture shining on the scarlet lips and on the red tongue as it lapped the white sharp teeth. Lower and lower went her head as the lips went below the range of my mouth and chin. . . . I could feel the soft, shivering touch of the lips on the super-sensitive skin of my throat, and the hard dents of two sharp teeth, just touching and pausing there. I closed my eyes in languorous ecstasy and waited—waited with beating heart.

Much later in the novel (Chapter 21), Dracula finally reaches his longed-for victim, Mina Harker, pulls open his shirt, opens a vein in his chest with his sharp fingernail, and then does the following:

> . . . his right hand gripped her by the back of the neck, forcing her face down on his bosom. Her white nightdress was

> smeared with blood, and a thin stream trickled down the man's bare breast which was shown by his torn-open dress. The attitude of the two had a terrible resemblance to a child forcing a kitten's nose into a saucer of milk to compel it to drink.

Because of the overt sexuality of the vampire myth, particularly as it was portrayed by Stoker, vampires began to arouse the interest of psychoanalysts. The psychoanalytic literature on the oral-sadistic and sexual aspects of *Dracula* and of vampires in general is varied, although Ernest Jones' treatment of the vampire in his book, *On the Nightmare* (1951), is the most often cited source of psychoanalytic speculation on the subject. More recent noteworthy additions to the literature are the contributions by Twitchell (1980), Roth (1977), Bierman, (1972) and Bentley (1972). Many of these essays can be found along with others in a collection of *Dracula* literary criticism by Carter (1988). For a Jungian literary interpretation, see the brief analysis put forth by Phillips (1986).

Author Stephen King has much to say on the subject of the sexuality of vampirism in his excellent survey of the horror genre, *Danse Macabre* (1981). In his discussion of *Dracula*, King (1981, p. 64) argues that ". . . much of the evil embodied in the Count is a perverse sexual evil. Stoker revitalized the vampire legend largely by writing a novel which fairly pants with sexual energy." Further, King astutely observes, "It is also sex without responsibility, and in the unique and amusing term coined by Erica Jong, the sex in *Dracula* can be seen as the ultimate zipless fuck" (p. 66). Interestingly, although King is often openly hostile to psychoanalytic speculation, he seems to be agreeing with Ernest Jones' interpretation of vampirism when he says, "The sexual basis of *Dracula* is an infantile oralism coupled with necrophilia. . . ." (p. 66). Presently, the erotic adventures of the vampire legend continue in the vampire novels of author Anne Rice (Ramsland, 1991).

CLINICAL VAMPIRISM (RENFIELD'S SYNDROME)

According to the legend of the vampire, it is really only after a vampire victim's first feeding, the first tasting of blood, that individuals cross over the line and become vampires. They then must forever serve the mad craving for blood that this experience initiates. This crossing over the line, the breach of a cultural taboo against the drinking of blood, is what marks the beginning of the disease of vampirism, both in legend and in fact. For this reason, the modern phenomenon called "clinical vampirism" is perhaps best understood in terms of the primitive theory of a disease caused by the violation of a taboo (see the introduction to this book). The excitement experienced by engaging in a forbidden act only reinforces the behavior and increases the likelihood that it will be repeated again and again.

Herschel Prins (1984), a British authority on clinical vampirism whose work has been invaluable in defining the syndrome, points out that in the psychiatric literature the word "vampirism" has been used to cover a spectrum of phenomena. Such rare activities as necrophagia (eating the flesh of the human dead), necrophilia (sexual excitement and contact with corpses), cannibalism, and other sequelae of a *lustmord* (lust-murder) such as necrosadism (the abuse of corpses) have been included under this label since the 19th century in addition to the traditional meaning of drinking the blood of others (vampirism) and one's own blood (autovampirism). All of these activities are discussed together in a paper on "unusual sexual syndromes" by Rebal, Faguet, and Woods (1982).

It is quite conceivable that Bram Stoker came into contact with the 1892 English translation of *Psychopathia Sexualis* (1886) by the famous German neurologist and psychiatrist Richard von Krafft-Ebing (1840–1902), which contains many vivid case histories of lust-murders involving necrophagia, necrophilia, blood drinking, and the sexual excitement that some individuals can only experience when they see fresh blood flowing, or imagine it to be doing so, from their sexual partners. The vampires in Stoker's book perform gruesome lust-murders on men, women, and even on children that are similar in tone to the graphic examples provided in Krafft-Ebing's famous text. The 19th century expert on sexual pathology defines "lust-murders" as "lust potentiated as cruelty, murderous lust extending to anthropophagy" (Krafft-Ebing, 1892, p. 62). The most vampire-like of the lust-murders cited by Krafft-Ebing is the often-cited story of a 19-year-old vinedresser by the name of Leger:

> Case 10. . . . . From youth moody, silent, shy of people. He starts out in search of a situation. He wanders about eight days in the forest, there catches a girl twelve years old, violates her,

> mutilates her genitals, tears out her heart, eats of it, drinks the blood, and buries the remains. (Krafft-Ebing, 1892, pp. 63–64)

The article by Prins in this collection includes his classification schema for the varying degrees of what he considers to be the best definition of vampirism. As he himself notes, it is based on the work of Bourguignon (1977; 1983). The model of clinical vampirism proposed here (and based on a reading of many of the case histories below) defines the syndrome according to a discernible course that fits all the case histories in one or more of its aspects. It is also proposed that the sexual blood-fetish syndrome defined here as clinical vampirism should bear a new eponymous label in future psychiatric treatments and be renamed Renfield's syndrome in honor of the character in Bram Stoker's *Dracula* who bore many of the classic signs and symptoms of the disorder.

The following are the proposed characteristics of Renfield's syndrome:

1. A pivotal event often leads to the development of vampirism (blood drinking). This usually occurs in childhood, and the experience of bleeding or the taste of blood is found to be "exciting." After puberty, this excitement associated with blood is experienced as sexual arousal.

2. The progression of Renfield's syndrome follows a typical course in many cases:

Autovampirism is generally developed first, usually in childhood, by initially self-inducing scrapes or cuts in the skin to produce blood, which is then ingested, to later learning how to open major blood vessels (veins, arteries) in order to drink a steady stream of warm blood more directly. The blood may then be ingested at the time of the opening, or may be saved in jars or other containers for later imbibing or for other reasons. Masturbation often accompanies autovampiristic practices.

Zoophagia (literally the eating of living creatures, but more specifically the drinking of their blood) may develop prior to autovampirism in some cases, but usually is next to develop. Persons with Renfield's syndrome may themselves catch and eat or drink the blood of living creatures such as insects, cats, dogs, or birds. The blood of other species may be obtained at places such as slaughter houses and then ingested. Sexual activity may or may not accompany these functions.

Vampirism in its true form is the next stage to develop—procuring and drinking the blood of living human beings. This may be done by stealing blood from hospitals, laboratories, and so forth, or by attempting to drink the blood directly from others. Usually this involves some sort of consensual sexual activity, but in lust-murder type cases and in other nonlethal violent crimes, the sexual activity and vampirism may not be consensual.

3. The compulsion to drink blood almost always has a strong sexual component associated with it.

4. Blood will sometimes take on an almost mystical significance as a sexualized symbol of life or power, and, as such, an experience of well-being or empowerment will be reported by those with Renfield's syndrome following such activities.

5. Persons with Renfield's syndrome are primarily male.

6. The defining characteristic of Renfield's syndrome is the blood-drinking compulsion. Other related activities such as necrophilia and necrophagia that do not have as their goal the drinking of blood are not to be considered aspects of this disorder.

THE RELEVANCE OF JUNG

Although C. G. Jung (1928/1966, p. 224) uses the word "vampire" only once in his entire 20-volume *corpus* of his *Collected Works* as a metaphor for the negative "animus possession" in a woman and negative "anima possession" in a man ("the woman's incubus consists of a host of masculine demons; the man's succubus is a vampire"), many scholars in the field of Renfield's syndrome have directly or indirectly cited his work as a possible source of interpretative material for the disorder. This acknowledgment is in recognition of the fact that vampirism combines both psychopathological and mythic elements that have an ancient tradition in the history of humankind, and that Jung's analytical psychology is very much concerned with the archaic vestiges of the human psyche. Bourguignon (1983) stresses the fact, for example, that vampirism is a clinical phenomenon in which myth, fantasy, and reality converge. Another authority, Prins (1984), openly speculates that "a Jungian conceptual framework might help us to link the two phenomena much more closely. It may be the case that some long-forgotten archetypal impulse may emerge and take control over an individual" (p. 292). One of the earliest (1964) and most comprehensively documented case histories (which is also included here) is that of R. S. McCully, who is in fact a Jungian analyst and who offers an amplification of the symbolism of vampirism using the literature of analytical psychology and mythology.

Although a detailed Jungian study devoted to the symbolism of blood drinking and vampirism is still lacking, just a few remarks here are offered as a starting point.

First, Jung mastered the ethnographic and anthropological literature of his time in order to document how even the psyche of the most civilized individual responded to life in ways directly analogous to the psychological processes of persons in primitive societies, and even went so far as to do make first-hand observations by conducting his own anthropological fieldwork in Africa and in the American southwest among the Pueblo Indians. Thus, the interpretation of vampirism in terms of the primitive concept of a disease caused and perpetuated by a breach of taboo would probably be congruent with his views. He would also no doubt agree with the anthropologist Sahlins' (1983, p. 88) observation that "cannibalism is always 'symbolic' even when it is real."

Second, Jung's psychology is derived from his lifelong research to construct a phenomenological taxonomy of human experience, and one of the most frequent motifs found through the ages and in the dreams and fantasies of his patients was that of a circular process, often symbolized by autophagous images analogous to the famous *uroborous*, the serpent that is constantly devouring its own tail and regenerating. In alchemical symbolism, this was known as the *circulatio*, the process by which a substance is heated in a reflux flask, with the resulting vapors rising and condensing, and then the condensed fluid feeding back into the belly of the flask where the whole process is repeated. The psychological process of distillation and refinement of psychic processes, then, was an autophagous one. Blood was a symbol of the *aqua permanens* (permanent water) of life and considered by the alchemists (the "adepts") as the seat of the soul; hence, Jung speculates as to whether certain recipes found in alchemical texts requiring admixtures of human blood are to be taken literally, and if so, whose blood was it? "Could it have been the adepts?" he wonders (Jung, 1955/1970, p. 485). Elsewhere (Jung 1942/1954/1969), in an essay on the "Transformation Symbolism in the Mass," Jung implicates the drinking of blood as a life-giving and mystical regenerative process in early Christian speculation that Jesus drank his own blood (p. 211).

In cases of Renfield's syndrome, then, the frequent reports of the nourishing or mystical life-enhancing quality of blood drinking may be, from a Jungian point of view, the behavioral expression of an instinctual drive within us all for continual psychological and physical replenishment with life-force (libido, energy) that usually only remains at the fantasy level—whether conscious or unconscious—and that has healing properties whose goal is the wholeness of the individual. This may also explain the intimate relationship of blood drinking to sexuality, the carnal expression of the life-force that Jung often called "the other face of God."

Interestingly, Jung did report a case of autovampirism without naming it as such. In a 1928 seminar on dream analysis (published for the first time in 1984), Jung comments on the mystical and redemptive symbolic significance of the act of drinking human blood, acknowledging that although such ideas were archaic and no longer widely believed at the level of collective consciousness, such a belief could still arise in individuals from time to time. As Jung relates the case history:

> A Swiss woman who came to me recently for treatment confessed after long resistances that she had a secret means to help her get to sleep, or to help against indigestion, etc: "An old man told me that secret. I drink the blood of Jesus. In the night, when I can't sleep, I repeat to myself: 'I am drinking the blood, drinking the blood of Jesus, the blood, the blood,' and then I feel myself drinking it and I can sleep. If I wake, I do it again—sometimes a dozen times a night." One day she went into the cellar—she was a very good housewife—and in standing on a chair to reach some apples on a shelf, she slipped and crashed down. She said: "I quickly drank the blood and was not hurt." She got a tremendous mystical association from drinking the blood; such things are still realities. (Jung, 1984, p. 36)

Third, the *pain* associated with the drawing of the blood is a symbolic spur to the further conscious development of the individual, as the assimilation of unconscious contents into consciousness can often only be accomplished through the anguish of inner conflict—a point that Jung often makes. An analogous activity that may be an external behavioral expression of the internal instinctual urge to further consciousness can be found among some persons who are severely or profoundly mentally retarded and who sometimes engage in self-injurious behaviors, including the eating of oneself. Clearly, the autophagous fantasy—of which vampirism is an expression—deserves further attention from psychologists, anthropologists, and other students of human life.

REFERENCES

Anglo, S. (1976). Melancholia and witchcraft: The debate between Weir, Bodin, and Scot. In *Folie et Déraison á la Renaissance*. Bruxelles.

Arens, W. (1979). *The Man-Eating Myth: Anthropology and Anthropophagy.* London: Oxford University Press.

Barber, P. (1988). *Vampires, Burial, and Death.* New Haven: Yale University Press.

Bentley, C. F. (1972). The monster in the bedroom: Sexual symbolism in Bram Stoker's *Dracula. Literature and Psychology*, 22, 27–34.

Bierman, J. S. (1972). *Dracula*: Prolonged childhood and illness and the oral triad. *American Imago*, 29, 186–198.

Bourguignon, A. (1972). Vampirism and autovampirism. *Annales Médico-Psychologiques*, *1*, 181–196.

Bourguignon, A. Vampirism and autovampirism. In Schlesinger, L. B., & Revitch, E. (Eds.) (1983). *Sexual Dynamics of Antisocial Behavior.* Springfield, IL: Charles C. Thomas.

Brown, P., & Tuzin, D. (Eds.) (1983). *The Ethnography of Cannibalism.* Washington, D.C.: The Society for Psychological Anthropology.

Carter, M. L. (1975). *Shadow of a Shade: A Survey of Vampirism in Literature.* New York: Gordon Press, 1975.

Carter, M. L. (1988). *Dracula: The Vampire and the Critics.* Ann Arbor: UMI Research Press.

Cohn, N. (1970). *The Pursuit of the Millennium: Revolutionary Millenarians and the Mystical Anarchists of the Middle Ages.* 2nd ed. New York: Oxford University Press.

Cohn, N. (1975). *Europe's Inner Demons: An Enquiry Inspired by the Great Witch Hunt.* New York: Basic Books.

Douglas, M. (Ed.) (1970). *Witchcraft Confessions and Accusations.* London: Tavistock.

Dresser, N. (1989). *American Vampires: Fans, Victims, Practitioners.* New York: W. W. Norton.

Florescu, R., & McNally, R. T. (1973). *Dracula: A Biography of Vlad the Impaler. 1431–1476.* New York: Hawthorn.

Florescu, R., & McNally, R. T. (1989). *Dracula: Prince of Many Faces.* New York: Little, Brown, & Co.

Gannaway, G. K. (1989). Historical truth versus narrative truth: Clarifying the role of exogenous trauma in the etiology of multiple personality disorder and its variants. *Dissociation, 2,* 205–220.

Goldstein, J. (1987). *Console and Classify: The French Psychiatric Profession in the Nineteenth Century..* Cambridge: Cambridge University Press.

Hicks, R. D. (1990). *In Pursuit of Satan: The Police and the Occult.* New York: Prometheus Books.

Hill, S., & Goodwin, J. (1989). Satanism: Similarities between patient accounts and pre-Inquisition historical sources. *Dissociation, 2,* 39–44.

Hock, S. (1901). *Die Vampyrsagen und ihre Verwertung in der deutschen Literatur.* Berlin.

Hogg, G. (1958). *Cannibalism and Human Sacrifice.* London: Kegan.

Hsia, R. P. (1988). *The Myth of Ritual Murder: Jews and Magic in Reformation Germany.* New Haven: Yale University Press.

James, E. O. (1933). *Origins of Sacrifice: A Study in Comparative Religion.* London: Routledge.

Jones, E. (1931/1951). *On the nightmare.* New York: Liveright.

Jung, C. G. (1929/1966). On the relations between the ego and the unconscious. In C. G. Jung, *Two Essays on Analytical Psychology. The Collected Works of C. G. Jung, Vol. 7.* Princeton: Princeton University Press.

Jung, C. G. (1969). Transformation symbolism in the Mass (1942/1954). In Jung, C. G., *Psychology and Religion: West and East. The Collected Works of C. G. Jung, Vol. 11.* Princeton: Princeton University Press.

Jung, C. G. (1970). *Mysterium Conjunctionis. The Collected Works of C. G. Jung, Vol. 14.* Princeton: Princeton University Press.

Jung, C. G. (1984). *Dream Analysis: Notes of the Seminar given in 1928–1930.* W. McGuire (Ed.). Princeton: Princeton University Press.

King, S. (1981). *Danse Macabre.* New York: Berkley.

Klaniczay, G. (1987). Decline of witches and rise of vampires in 18th century Hapsburg monarchy. *Ethnologica Europea, 17,* 165–180.

Klaniczay, G. (1990). *The Uses of Supernatural Power: The Transformation of Popular Religion in Medieval and Early-Modern Europe.* Princeton: Princeton University Press.

Krafft-Ebing, R. (1892). *Psychopathia Sexualis, with special reference to contrary sexual instinct: A medico-legal study.* C. G. Chaddock, trans. Philadelphia: F. A. Davis.

Lanning, K. (1989, Oct.). Satanic, occult, ritualistic crime: A law enforcement perspective. *The Police Chief,* pp. 1–11.

Lanning, K. V. (1991). Ritual abuse: A law enforcement perspective. *Child Abuse and Neglect, 15,* 171–173.

Leatherdale, C. (Ed.) (1987). *The Origins of Dracula.* London: William Kimber.

Lewis, I. M. (1986). The cannibal's cauldron. In, I. M. Lewis (Ed.), *Religion in Context: Cults and Charisma*. Cambridge: Cambridge University Press.

Lipschiltz, L. (1882). *Christliche Zeugnisse gegen die Blutschuldigung der Juden*. Berlin.

Ludlam, H. (1962). *A Biography of Dracula: The Life Story of Bram Stoker*. London: W. Foulsham.

McNally, R. T. (1983). *Dracula Was a Woman: In Search of the Blood Countess of Transylvania*. New York: McGraw-Hill.

McNally, R. T., & Florescu, R. (1972). *In Search of Dracula: A True History of Dracula and the Vampire Legends*. Greenwich, CT: New York Graphic Society.

Nöll, R. (1989). Satanism, UFO abductions, historians and clinicians: Those who do not remember the past. . . . *Dissociation*, 2, 251–253.

Noll, R. (In press). Devil-worshippers and satanists in Old Europe and in the New World: A brief historical survey. In G. Fraser (Ed.), Satanic Ritual Abuse. Washington, D.C.: American Psychiatric Press.

Phillips, R. (1986). The agony and the ecstasy: A Jungian analysis of two vampire novels, Meredith Ann Pierce's *The Darkangel* and Bram Stoker's *Dracula*. *West Virginia University Philological Papers, 31*, 10–19.

Prins, H. (1984). Vampirism—Legendary or clinical phenomenon? *Medicine, Science, and the Law, 24*, 283–293.

Putnam, F. W. (1991). The satanic ritual abuse controversy. *Child Abuse and Neglect, 15*, 175–179.

Ramsland, K. (1991). *Anne Rice: Prism of the Night*. New York: New American Library.

Rebal, R. F., Faguet, R. A., & Woods, S. M. (1982). Unusual sexual syndromes. In C. T. H. Friedmann & R. A. Faguet (Eds.), *Extraordinary Disorders of Human Behavior*. New York: Plenum Press.

Resch, A. (1901). *Siebenbürgische Münzen und Medaillen von 1538 bis zur Gegenwart*. Hermannstadt: Verein Für Siebenbürgische Landeskunde.

Roth, C. (Ed.) (1934). *The Ritual Murder Libel and the Jew: Report by Cardinal Lorenzo Ganganelli (Pope Clement XIV)*. London.

Roth, P. A. (1977). Suddenly sexual women in Bram Stoker's *Dracula*. *Literature and Psychology*, 27, 113.

Roth, P. A. (1982). *Bram Stoker*. Boston: Twayne.

Russell, J. B. (1990, Nov.). Personal communication.

Sahlins, M. (1983). Raw women, cooked men and other 'great things' of the Fiji Islands. In P. Brown & D. Tuzin (Eds.), *The Ethnography of Cannibalism*. Washington, D.C.: The Society for Psychological Anthropology.

Stevens, P. (1989) Satanism: Where are the folklorists? *New York Folklore, 15*, 1–22.

Stoker, B. (1897). *Dracula*. London: Constable.

Stoker, B. Original foundation notes and data for *Dracula*. In the collection of the Philip H. and A. S. W. Rosenbach Foundation, Philadelphia. (An edited reproduction with commentary by J. S. Bierman is in preparation for publication.)

Strack, H. L. (1909). *The Jew and Human Sacrifice*. H. Blanchamp, trans. New York.

Summers, M. (1928). *The Vampire: His Kith and Kin*. London: Headley Bros.

Summers, M. (1928). *The Vampire: His Kith and Kin.* London: Headley Bros.

Summers, M. (1929). *The Vampire in Europe.* London: Headley Bros.

Tannahill, R. (1975). *Flesh and Blood: A History of the Cannibal Complex.* New York: Stein & Day.

Trachtenberg, J. (1943). *The Devil and the Jews: The Medieval Conception of the Jew and its Relation to Modern Antisemitism.* New Haven: Yale University Press.

Twitchell, J. B. (1980). The vampire myth. *American Imago,* 83–92.

Van Benschoten, S. C. (1990). Multiple personality disorder and satanic ritual abuse: The issue of credibility. *Dissociation, 3,* 22–30.

Victor, J. S. (1989). A rumor-panic about a dangerous satanic cult in Western New York. *New York Folklore, 15,* 23–49.

Victor, J. S. (1990). Satanic cult rumors as a contemporary legend. *Western Folklore,* Special Issue: Contemporary Legends in Emergence, (Spring–Summer).

1

Vampirism

A Review with New Observations

RICHARD L. VANDEN BERGH, *M.D.*[1]
JOHN F. KELLY, *M.D.*

Vampirism is defined as the act of drawing blood from an object, (usually a love object) and receiving resultant sexual excitement and pleasure. The blood may be drawn by various means such as biting, cutting, etc. The sucking or drinking of the blood from the wound is often an important part of the act but not an essential one. Vampirism is not considered in this paper as a sexual desire for corpses, as it has sometimes been defined. This latter syndrome is better classified as necrophilia.

The scientific literature on the subject of vampirism is extremely meager. What references there are, for the most part, treat the subject briefly and superficially. But the authors feel that such behavior and fantasies are more common and important than their relative absence in the literature would suggest. For though it is true that cases of pure vampirism are relatively rare, it is also true that vampiristic content, wishes, and fantasies often are seen as reaction formations or sublimations. Not as well camouflaged, they frequently appear in dreams.

[1]University of Colorado Medical Center, Denver

Reprinted with permission from *Archives of General Psychiatry*, 1964, Vol. 11, 543–547.

Fenichel, in his book on the *Psychoanalytic Theory of Neurosis*, while discussing infantile sexuality notes how "often oral sadistic sucking fantasies directed against objects can be observed," and he uses the word vampire in this regard.[1] Any psychiatrist who has worked extensively with psychotics has seen such fantasies and behavior in his patients.

For these reasons it was felt that a more comprehensive study and review of the subject was indicated and might be helpful in stimulating further interest.

By way of introduction it is worthy of note that if one accepts the myths and legends of the past as having had psychological factors as the causal basis of their existence, then the universality of the legend of the vampire has importance. Though these legendary figures performed acts besides those included within the bounds of our definition, (such as returning from the dead) nonetheless the biting of the object and sucking of its blood was a most essential element. These legends can be found as early as Greek and Roman mythology and were seen throughout Europe, Asia, and parts of Africa.[4]

Turning to the early literature related to the subject Havelock Ellis, in 1903, writes at some length of the "love-bite," telling first of its frequency "in the literature of ancient as well as of modern times in the East as well as in the West." Later he adds that:

> The result of the love-bite in its extreme form is to shed blood. This cannot be regarded as the direct aim of the bite in its normal manifestations, for the mingled feelings of close contact, of passionate gripping, of symbolic devouring, which constitute the emotional accompaniments of the bite would be too violently discomposed by actual wounding and real shedding of blood. With some persons, however, perhaps more especially women, the love-bite is really associated with a conscious desire, even if more or less restrained, to draw blood, a real delight in this process, a love of blood. Probably this only occurs in persons who are not absolutely normal, but on the borderline of the abnormal. . . . There is scarcely any natural object with so profoundly emotional an effect as blood. . . . Normally the fascination of blood, if present at all during sexual excitement, remains more or less latent, either because it is weak or because the checks that inhibit it are inevitably

> very powerful. Occasionally it becomes more clearly manifest, and this may happen early in life.[3]

Ellis then cites a few clinical examples of patients who at a young age experienced sexual stimulation at the sight of blood. Among them he describes a girl who as a child was very fond of watching dog fights especially if much blood was shed during the fight. Later in life she frequently cut or scratched herself to see and suck the blood thinking the taste delicious. This produced strong sexual feelings and often orgasm, especially if at the time she fantasied sucking the blood of some attractive man. She also carried out these urges in her relationship with her husband. On several occasions she bit him until the blood came and then sucked the blood during coitus.

Dr. Von Krafft-Ebing, in 1892, cites the case of "a married man (who) presented himself with numerous scars or cuts on his arms." He told their origin as follows: "When he wished to approach his wife, who was young and somewhat 'nervous,' he first had to make a cut in his arm. Then she would suck the wound and during the act become violently excited sexually." He makes only the following notation in the case. "This case recalls the widespread legend of the vampires, the origin of which may perhaps be referred to such sadistic facts."[6]

Of the lay literature, the Marquis de Sade's famous novels are worthy of mention. In these the heroes often plan scenes of debauchery in which the flowing of blood is an essential element of coitus.

Turning to the more recent psychiatric literature on the subject; in 1957, London describes a case of Nymphomania and Vampirism. A female patient who "during the acme of excitement bites her lover on the neck and shoulders, often drawing blood."[7] In describing another case, he mentioned a female patient who:

> discovered that she became sexually excited by biting her roommate on the neck and shoulders during mutual masturbation. She liked to bite and suck the flesh until she was able to produce a red spot on her partner's body (ecchymosis). On one occasion her girl friend cut herself while opening a can of vegetables. She went over and sucked the blood from the bleeding finger, telling her friend that her saliva was antiseptic and would heal the wound. The evidence tends to support the existence of sexual excitement associated with this pecu-

liar deviation known as vampirism,—(blood sucking). She reports that she felt a sensation in her vagina as she tasted the blood of her friend's finger. . . . [8]

REPORT OF CASES

Two cases from the authors' own experience are now described as follows:

Case 1.

Case 1 was a 28-year-old patient, the eldest of three siblings. His birth and early development were essentially normal, except that his mother was periodically ill so that he and the other children were raised by a series of governesses. At approximately 8 years of age he unconsciously produced a series of nose bleeds by picking at the inside of his nose. On one of these occasions he remembered consciously having a feeling of pleasure and being "excited" by the sight of the blood dripping on to the floor. At age 11, he became a rabid collector of toy pistols, having a definite preference for the larger, longer, and more powerful ones. At age 12, he reached puberty and almost simultaneously developed his vampiristic tendencies. He found erotic satisfaction by nicking a vein in his arm and watching the blood flow from it. Simultaneously he would masturbate and fantasize. His fantasies were usually of puncturing the neck vessels of an adolescent youth with a smooth skin and a thin, long neck with prominent vessels. Occasionally instead of fantasizing he would read vampire stories. Whenever he reached an orgasm, he would shut off the bleeding. These acts were always performed in secret. He would catch the blood in bottles or glass jars, later throwing it away, but occasionally keeping it and drinking it, receiving pleasure and excitement while doing so. With time he changed and improved his technique, moving from veins in his arms to the arteries, and later still, to the arteries in his neck. The blood spurting from the arteries with rhythmic pulsation greatly enhanced his sexual pleasure. Finally he was able to manipulate the blood from the artery in a direct stream into his mouth. This he did in the shower where any spillage of blood would be quickly washed down the drain and therefore remain undetected. There was no awareness of any element of pain involved. He would occasionally wrestle with boys in such a way as to get his mouth into direct contact with the other boy's neck. However, he always maintained sufficient control of his impulses so as to never fully act them out. At age 14, he became keenly interested in real guns, but during that year accidentally shot and wounded a friend. Under the stress of the situation, his episodes of blood letting greatly increased in frequency, leading shortly to the development of an iron-deficiency anemia. This was medically treated without the patient revealing his secret. At age 22, under the stress of involvement in a car accident, necessitating a subsequent appearance in court, the blood letting again greatly increased followed immediately by the appearance of left-sided weakness. This, however, quickly resolved with the cessation of the blood letting. But two months later, on this occasion under the stress of college examinations, the blood letting again increased and a second episode of mild left hemiparesis occurred. This again resolved itself with cessation of the blood-letting. At age 23, again under the stress of examinations, the left-sided hemiparesis briefly recurred. In the ensuing months the patient's ego control steadily decreased, culminating in a schizophrenic break with immediate hospitalization.

Case 2.

Case 2 was a 20-year-old white male examined in the setting of a prison where he was serving a sentence for automobile theft. It was brought to the attention of the prison authorities that several of the more aggressive homosexual inmates of the institution were stealing iron tablets, and at the same time expressing fears of developing anemia. Investigation revealed that the patient was trading homosexual favors with these inmates in return for the opportunity of sucking their blood. Little factual information on the patient's birth and early development could be obtained. The younger of two brothers, he had little contact with his sibling, however, as the latter was sentenced to a reformatory and left the parental home at a very young age. The patient's earliest memory, at approximately 5 years of age, was one of his mother holding his right hand over an open stove burner as a form of punishment. Though he related the memory as a painful one, he did so with a somewhat inappropriate pleasurable affect. The patient's father was described as being "drunk most of the time," on which occasions he was abusive and cruel to the patient. On several occasions the patient was beaten by his father until he was bloodied, and on one occasion switched by his mother until his legs were bleeding. His first memory of a feeling of excitement at the sight of blood was stimulated by seeing dogs which had been run over by cars in the street. During his late childhood, he put his hands in the blood of a dog so killed, tasted the blood, and felt definite sexual excitement. His parents frequently fought each other physically and when he began masturbating his fantasies included these parental battles and the blood of the killed dogs. At approximately the age of 11, he was introduced into mutual masturbation by an older boy and again fantasied the brutal and bloody fights of his parents, as well as seeing his partner "bleed somehow." At age 14 he first had heterosexual intercourse with a girl four years his elder. He obtained his greatest pleasure from this experience, by sucking on her breasts and neck, producing areas of reddening. Later his masturbatory fantasies included "letting the blood out" of these reddened areas. At approximately the same time, the patient began displaying antisocial tendencies. During the next few years these included petty thievery, breaking of probation, suspicion of car theft, and jail sentences for vagrancy, culminating in his being sentenced to prison, as previously stated. During those years he had numerous abnormal sexual contacts. The first occurred when he was 15. "Picked up" in a movie theatre by an older homosexual the patient indulged in mutual fellatio with the man and was able to persuade him to allow the patient to cut his chest and neck in order to "see the blood." When this happened the patient became quite

> excited and began sucking the blood. He experienced a feeling of becoming quite "powerful" and quickly reached a climax. From then on his primary sexual aim was for this activity with both men and women. He discovered that it was easier to obtain this from homosexuals, in return for their receiving homosexual favors from him. He used the veins of his "victims" because "I could get more blood that way." These were usually in the antecubital fossa, and usually around the area of the neck. Though he frequently wished to obtain the blood from the area of the groin the patient never found partners willing to allow him to do this. During such activity he would almost always experience an erection and subsequent ejaculation. Just prior to his admission to the institution where he was evaluated, he was reported to have undergone an overt psychotic episode. The records of this, however, were inadequate. Nonetheless the overall impression was that this patient was schizophrenic though not actively psychotic at the time of evaluation.

Previous publications on vampirism have stated that the dynamics involved probably fall under the heading of oral sadism. Fenichel's quotation on the subject has already been noted. London, (as another example), states "both cannibalistic traits and vampirism may be classified as forms of oral sadism in contrast to other forms of sadism (urethral and anal)."[8]

Certainly many of the cases reported and seen would tend clearly to support this view. Karpman for example cites the following case of a vampiristic fantasy.

> The patient asked herself anxiously what she might do if a young girl came into her power, docile and willing to submit. She said: "I would like most of all to kiss her breasts, then tear or bite them off and eat them. I would tear out the vagina, the uterus and the rectum. I would eat all of them and with them the inner portion of the thigh which borders on the sexual parts. . . . I would at last find my way to the heart and then drink the heart's blood, then pluck out the heart and perhaps eat it."[5]

Nacht and his co-workers under the heading of sado masochistic perversions discuss the case of a murderer whom they had been able to observe, though not to psychoanalyze.

> During the 1914–1918 war he was a stretcher bearer and loved to feel the blood of the wounded drench his clothes and to wear for a long time afterwards underclothing stiffened by the blood. Following this he had taken the habit of going regularly to slaughter houses to drink a glass of warm blood which, according to him, was a therapeutic measure, for he had hypochondrical tendencies.

Previously the patient had murdered a female companion. An unpremeditated murder, followed by a frenzied cutting up, evisceration, cannibalism, and orgasm. Nacht felt that the "acting out of oral aggression was able to go so far as cannibalism and to manifest itself in a chronic state by the degraded need to drink blood at slaughter houses (this without any orgasms)."[9]

These two latter cases show clearly the oral sadistic elements in the dynamics of the syndrome. However, this does not appear to be true of all cases. A closer look at some cases reveals that often the element of sadism, in the true analytic sense of the word, plays only a minor role, or occasionally is not clearly discernible at all. The wound in such cases is not inflicted by the patient, nor is there an element of pain present. This is exemplified in the second case cited by the authors. There the patient's homosexual victims in the prison often reported a sensation of pleasure and a total absence of any pain and the wounds were often self-inflicted by them without any participation on the part of the patient.

In other cases, though symptoms of orality are present, much of the pathology appears to be at a later stage of libidinal development. An important clue to this, and a factor playing a more major role than it has previously been given credit for, is the symbolic meaning of the blood itself. For instance an insufficient explanation is given in the case cited by Nacht as to why the patient should have derived such pleasure from feeling the "blood of the wounded drench his clothes," and from wearing underclothes for a long time afterwards "stiffened by the blood." A similar incomplete explanation as to the role played by the blood is apparent in many cases. The authors feel, however, that the symbolism of the blood is a most important factor, which in all likelihood varies from case to case. In the first case cited by the authors, the early stages of intensive psychotherapy revealed that the blood symbolized to the patient, "an unobtainable object," or "forbidden fruit," which, as his therapy progressed, proved to be his "unobtainable" and "forbidden" oedipal wishes toward his mother. By the letting of the blood he was symbolically obtaining the "unobtainable Mother," and as this symbolic blood rhythmically spurted from a lacerated artery his sexual excitement rose to the point of orgasm. Though symptoms of orality were obviously present, his unresolved oedipal wishes were clearly manifested and it was to this latter level of his development that he primarily regressed under stress. Poor masculine identification during the oedipal years, due both to his father's frequent absence from the home, and subtle unconscious seductive behavior on the part of his mother, led to his homosexual tendencies.

In the second case cited by the authors the patient left the institution before a truly adequate study could be completed. However, certain probable, but none the less theoretical, impressions were obtained. When discussing his feelings concerning the drinking of the blood, the patient stated that it was warm and "tasted rich," that it somehow gave him a feeling of well being, and that it gave him a feeling of being "powerful, like I had taken something powerful from them." It seems most likely, although obvious symptoms of oral fixation are again present, that the incorporation of blood symbolized to him a powerful and highly sexualized incorporation. He seemed to equate sexual union with this incorporation of "powerful juices." These factors coupled with the extraordinary degree to which the patient intertwined sexuality with all his aggressive sadistic acts, the parental history of physical combat, and the masturbatory fantasies centered around these fights, all pointed to a major fixation around the oedipal level of development.

Indications are also seen in many cases, that the letting of blood symbolizes various unconscious aggressive hostile wishes including murder. Fleiss in discussing the case of "Little Hans" has introduced the idea of the importance of quantitatively small flows of blood. He suggests that when the bleeding is limited in fact or fantasy it may be a typical element in the primal fantasy of castration. He cites several examples to support the possible validity of his hypothesis. Then he concludes with a question; "One wonders is the limitation of bleeding a mark, distinguishing castration from murder?"[2]

In conclusion the authors wish to stress the following points. The syndrome and fantasies of vampirism are more frequent and important than their relative absence in the literature would suggest. The specific symptoms seen in vampirism have their dynamic basis not only in the unresolved conflicts at the oral sadistic level, but at other levels of libidinal development as well. Examples of this were given in the two cases cited by the authors. The symbolic representation of the blood should always be investigated as an important clue to the better understanding of the underlying pathology. Oedipal wishes, fear of castration, and aggressive hostile wishes, are examples of these many various unresolved conflicts which can be symbolized in the patients' minds by the blood.

REFERENCES

1. Fenichel, O.: Psychoanalytic Theory of Neuroses, ed 1, New York: W. W. Norton, Co., Inc., 1945, p. 65.
2. Fliess, R.: Erogencity and Libido, New York: International Universities Press Inc., 1956, pp. 30–31.
3. Ellis, H.: Studies in Psychology of Sex, ed. 2, Philadelphia: F. A. Davis Company, 1927, vol. 3, pp. 84, 120–123.
4. Jones, E.: On Nightmare, ed. 2, New York: Liveright Publishing Co., 1951, pp. 98–130.
5. Karpman, D.: Obsessive Paraphilias (Perversions), Arch Neurol Psychiat 32:604–605 (Sept) 1934.
6. Von Krafft-Ebing, R.: Psychopathia Sexualis, ed. 7, Philadelphia: F. A. Davis Company, 1895, p. 81.
7. London, L. S.: Sexual Deviations in Female, revised edition, New York: Julian Press Inc., 1957, p. 123.
8. London, L. A., and Caprio, F. S.: Sexual Deviations, Washington: Linacre Press, 1958, pp. 603–604.
9. Nacht, S.; Diatkine, R.; and Favreau, J.: Ego in Perverse Relationships, Int Psychoanal 37: 406–407, 1956.

2

Vampirism

Historical Perspective and Underlying Process in Relation to a Case of Auto-Vampirism

ROBERT S. McCULLY, *Ph.D.*[1]

The vampire has been a subject in folk tale, superstition and myth throughout the history of man. Since it is generally thought to be a predominately Slavic myth, and its pervasive recurrence in history is seldom recognized, some attention to the historical perspective of the vampire image may be useful.

Some of the most venerable members of the pantheon of human gods were given to blood sucking in one form or another. However, the symbolism of the act may have no connection with vampirism *per se*. For example, a whole group of Vajra deities in Tibetan Lamaism are represented as blood drinkers, but their dripping flagons of blood merely symbolize the need for mastery over life. Yet, in the Gilgamesh legend, the oldest in recorded history, the vampire theme emerged and its qual-

[1]Payne Whitney Psychiatric Clinic, The New York Hospital; Cornell University Medical College.

Reprinted with permission from *Journal of Nervous and Mental Disease*, 1964, Vol. 139, 440–452.

ities were as clearly described and gory as those of medieval times. The earliest known depiction of a vampire appears on a prehistoric Assyrian bowl, and shows a man copulating with a vampire whose head has been severed from her body (11, p. 226). In India, the vampire theme can be traced to the Atharva Veda, and the *Baital-Pachisi, or Tales of a Vampire*, form an important part of the body of ancient literary heritage. In ancient Mexico, vampires were called Ciuateteo, and were associated with women who had died in their first labor. The Chinese vampire, Ch'ing Shih, often described in stories of the T'ang Dynasty, takes origin from much earlier times, and has a close similarity with the vampire image of the West. It would appear that a psychic counterpart necessary for projection of the vampire into myth has existed since earliest times, and that it may be among the most archaic images known.

Joseph Campbell (1, pp. 833–863) has stated that European mythology and folk tale suffered from a comparative poverty until around the twelfth century, when works of Indian, Celtic and Arabian masters of narrative found their way onto the European scene. Some of the most beautiful of the European tales can be traced to Eastern and Celtic sources. Indian story forms influenced the style and content of the works of Boccaccio and Chaucer. The vampire theme may have reached Western Europe through Turkey and the Balkans, having come from India.

The vampire theme caught the imagination of a number of the most influential literary minds of the past century. Goethe, Southey, Byron and Baudelaire wrote about the subject, and it played an important role in John Keats' *Lamia*, and in Samuel Taylor Coleridge's *Christobel*. In *Justine*, the Marquis de Sade vividly depicted a character who takes lustful pleasure in watching the blood flow from the veins of his victims. Le Fanu and Thomas Preskett Prest were among those who brought the image to the popular press, while Bram Stoker's *Dracula* made the vampire a household word. Even so brilliant a scientific mind as that of James Clerk Maxwell was fascinated with the image and he wrote a poem, *The Vampyre*, in his fourteenth year.

Ernest Jones (3, p. 99) described the vampire as "a nocturnal spirit who embraces a sleeper to suck his blood from him; he is evidently a product of the nightmare." Jones (3, pp. 98–130) discussed vampirism as a symbolic manifestation and, using the psychoanalytic point of view, he has described and drawn together considerable information about the vampire myth in Eastern Europe. In his review of writings on the subject, he indicated that certain popularized figures described in the annals of sexual criminology as "vampires" were necrophiliacs. Several sensational accounts of criminal psychopaths in Europe in the nineteenth and twentieth centuries were mistakenly called "vampires." The *Encyclopedie Medico-Chirurgicale* records that Epaulard (1901) published a thesis, entitled *Vampirisme*, written at Lyons in France. These case histories dealt mainly with criminal psychopaths and necrophilia, however, and may not be directly pertinent to the subject of this study.

This paper is concerned with a subject who showed overt vampiristic characteristics. This uniquely pathological drive was acted out on himself, while a similar drive toward others was partly contained. There is no parallel case recorded in the literature. When discussed at all, the notion of vampirism has been regarded as a theme in mythology derived from dream or fantasy (2, p. 65; p. 489).

The purpose of this paper is to offer some information about the nature and origin of the vampire image and to relate this information to the subject of the study. The subject was studied in depth by a variety of projective techniques, and the findings will be reported and discussed. Some light may thus be thrown on the dynamics of the individual subject, and the findings may offer material for speculation about possible theoretical correlates.

CASE MATERIAL

The subject was a young adult, unmarried, white male patient. In order to protect the privacy of the patient, no details other than those descriptive of his symptoms will be included. No known factors in his background would connect him with any special attitudes or exposure to the vampire myth. His earliest memories (age three) included having seen a dog which had been hit by a car lying in a pool of blood and, while sitting on a child's toilet, having had his brother squirt water from a syringe at him through the keyhole. At four, he remembered having had a nurse place his cold hands on her neck after a winter's walk in the park. There were no unusual childhood diseases. Masturbation began at age 11, and became associated with drawing his own blood and a compulsion to see it. He achieved this by puncturing his neck veins, and by performing the Valsalva maneuver, he could make the blood pour rapidly while watching in a mirror. In time, he learned to obtain arterial blood from his neck, having used a broken razor to puncture first a small artery, and later the common carotid artery. He discovered that by lying on his back, he could catch the spray of blood in his mouth and drink it. At times, a cup was used. Later, he learned to puncture the basilic vein in his arm and suck the blood directly. Masturbation began after having started the bloodletting, and reached ejaculation. This was accompanied by fantasies of taking blood from a young, smooth, hairless boy with prominent neck arteries. There was no fantasy of other young boys' genitals, and the subjects of fantasy were never female. The frequency of these episodes was about once every three weeks. Masturbation itself was much more frequent, and was accompanied by fantasies of sucking blood from the necks of young boys. During one period of adolescence, he found a young boy who would allow him to put his mouth on his neck for a short time.

He was known to have a congenital vascular anomaly of the right cerebral hemisphere. This came to light in relation to the appearance of partial paralysis (not long before his hospitalization). There were complicating hysterical features as well, and he made use of his physical handicap for purposes of secondary gain. The latter may be observed in the language used and in his approach to the Rorschach. During a period of hospitalization, he showed a curious, unexplained cyclic mood-swing which was not due to medication. For some time, he showed a four-day period of elation, followed by twelve days of depression. This repeated itself for a period, but was not characteristic of the entire period of hospitalization (one year). He said that he noticed his deepest depression coincided with the appearance of the full moon. He reported not infrequent dreams of bloodletting, which created a pleasant feeling at the time, but that he felt anxiety upon awakening. At least one known attempt to puncture the common carotid artery was made during his stay at the hospital. When describing his subjective attitudes during the blood-letting episodes, he reported that at one time he would feel a sense of peace as if being loved by someone, while at another time, he felt as if he had subdued somebody who had attacked him.

Except for periods of elation, a sustained depressed mood was obvious during his hospitalization. There was no history of either heterosexual or homosexual experiences, nor of any use of alcohol or tobacco. He was well aware of the abnormality of his behavior.

Projective Materials

A variety of projective stimuli was used. These included the Rorschach, a drawing series (human figures, animal and tree), Miale-Holsopple Sentence-Completion, a specially devised word-association test, Bender-Gestalt, projective questions and handwriting sample. The Rorschach materials were as follows:

RORSCHACH[2]

RESPONSE	INQUIRY
	Card II
1) 16″. That's a little more difficult, it looks almost like something anatomical, curious looking. I just don't know what to think on this. First impression was not quite so immediate, it did have some sort of facial appearance, but then the red parts of it changed that feeling I've had. I never had any kind of test like this before. [Say whatever occurs to you.] Well, I suppose you are supposed to report some kind of sensation or impression, and that's hard for me to do. W F(CF, Fm) At	1) Lower part of anatomy of some large animal. [Q] Overall shape, part of a living thing, or once part of a living thing. Color disrupts that, originally the color made it harder to decide what it is. The red could be blood that came from it, ripped out or dissected, and red is blood that came out. This is not new, a second look at it, oozing out, and a drawing, the red looks like a fluid and it drained symmetrically.
2) Some kind of face. [Q] Looks sort of like a skull a little bit, as did the other. The red suggested something anatomical, something dissected out of an animal. Pelvis keeps popping in my mind, animal pelvis, but I guess it shouldn't. W F At	2) I was cheating a little. [Meaning cuts of all red] I'd like to turn it, [v] now more like a skull with top part removed.

[2] Only those responses referred to in this text.

RESPONSE	INQUIRY
Card IV	
1) 6″. Another strange one. Kelp you see in shallows, salt harbors, but so symmetrical. Does look like seaweed, but that's not helpful, I suppose. DW cF O tendency	1) This curved thing with its shading made it look like Northern lights (female area at top). A curtain-like effect, illustration, fold effect, kaleidoscopic color effect. The shading makes it look like that—that give the effect, shading gives translucency. It looks translucent and like a fold. Shading.
Card VIII	
1) 18″. Oh, we got colors this time, sort of bilious colors too. Looks like a couple of salamanders or frogs, tearing a piece of water vegetation as might be seen under water. Color scheme is interesting—on either side of the symmetrical axis of symmetry, each animal comes out of an orange area and is surrounded by pinkish area same color, and are touching green, blue-green projections with one foot and touching grey-blue-green with other leg, and other hind leg is more purple. I'm just describing the way it's designed, that's wasting it, but I don't know what else to do. Maybe I'd get better with some years. W FM(CF,F/C) A P tendency.	1) [Q-salamander] Fish-shaped, don't know what. [Q-color] Yes, somewhat. [Q-underwater] Color scheme.

LIMITS

[Patient was asked to look through the cards and see if anything reminded him of people. He took this quite literally and spent a great deal of time on each card.]

Card I: This looks like a witch-like person, creature perched on a rock, being reflected from a still pool. (Side D)—hat, cape is projection, and bottom is cloak. Projections look like hands pointing—part of the witch. Still looks like a fox face though.

Card IV: This one, only thing here—this looks like a heavy man in overcoat with pack on his back, stooping under the weight of the load. He's carrying a cane or umbrella, it sticks out in front, but doesn't look right since nothing sticks out in back of him. It occurs to me, looks like an angel, mythical figure, looking down at a tome or book—or a witch with pointed cap with object in his hands, a winged being of some kind.

Card VI: Here again, this projection looks like somebody bending over with a heavy load on his back. [Q-kind of person] Heavily clothed. Two of them of course, one on each side. The Ghost of Christmas Past, from Charles Dickens. Looks like he, or it, is carrying some kind of burden on his shoulder or back, and a great big cloak spreading around on the ground.

Neither the Rorschach responses nor any of the other projective methods contained evidence for schizophrenic involvement *per se*. Twice on the Rorschach, his associations had an autistic quality, but in both cases, they were offered more as asides than as having to do with the basic image he had produced. Still, the nature of these associations raised the question of near-contamination (in which unrelated images fuse at the expense of logic), and hence suggested the possibility of underlying schizophrenic features.

Instead of containing bizarre ideas or a welter of autistic material, the projective findings were characterized by extensive evidence for depression throughout and a pervasive lack of emotional development. At times, he showed a surprising degree of adaptiveness, while at others, raw lack of adaptiveness showed through. His emotional development was so primitive that one may consider him virtually unformed in both the emotional and psychosexual spheres. On the other hand, his intellectual development had been appropriate to both his age and his excellent potential. The contrast between development in his intellectual and emotional worlds was profound.

In his approach to the Rorschach, there was a perplexity and verbalized ideational impotency that could be associated with organic qualities, like those appearing when an individual feels the loss of intellectual ability and the personality mobilizes itself in face of the threat. These qualities were difficult to evaluate in this subject, however, because of his constant complaints about "loss of ability" when none had been demonstrated, and because of the certainty of secondary gain. At the same time, he was known to have organic concomitants. He could demonstrate a remarkable, if highly circumstantial memory, and he showed perfect recall of the Bender designs. It was doubtful that any intellectual loss due to CNS pathology was present.

The language of the Rorschach showed how circumstantial and defended he was. He often set up high standards of perfection for himself that he assured himself of defeat. A strong obsessive-compulsive patterning was obvious throughout all he did. There were signs of some decompensation within that defense system, though these were not extensive.

By and large, all of the projective stimuli primarily reflected his defensive facade. At all times, he operated as if he had to keep himself in a tight, compulsive strait jacket, and to get out of it would invite chaos. It was as if he could move with others only intellectually, and the moment he stopped intellection, he was unrelated to others.

Implicit within some of the materials was an almost obsessive need to keep absolute separation between actual experiences and what had not yet been experienced. One may observe in the Rorschach materials how vague and uncommitted he was about his reactions to Card II, but then, as if drawn along by momentum and in spite of himself, something formless, but raw and primitive, emerged by the end of the inquiry about the card. His remarks about the color of the card were provocative. One was reminded here of his earliest memory, that of the dog in the pool of blood. He not only stated that the red color represented blood, but made a judgment about its freshness. It was blood that disrupted the possibility of *life* in the image. Here the subject's own association linked his bizarre need with a concrete struggle between life and death. This may remove the matter from the narrower context of sex into the basic struggle for existence. This is, of course, the basic motive in the vampire. The need for renewal of life is concretized by extracting it from others. It should be remembered that the subject was not at all unaware of the morbidity of his behavior and desires, and he viewed the matter rather like having been caught in the web of a terrible curse. His choice for the animal he would like most to be was interesting in this regard. He wrote, "What occurs to me is not really an animal, but something that flies, maybe a hawk or a bird of prey, or better, an albatross." He has acted out on himself bizarre needs, and while he wished to, he dared not act them out on others. Even though he identified with the sado-masochistic impulse, as shown by the bird of prey, he clung to hope with the image of good omen, the albatross. Still, while restraining his desires toward others, he was like the bird of Coleridge's poem, "It ate the food it ne'er had eat." This kinship with the mood of *The Rime of the Ancient Mariner* will be taken up later.

As far as can be seen from the projective materials, the subject's dynamics centered around an enormously undifferentiated passivity. That the need simply to "suck" could become connected with sadistic impulses may be supported by the primitive qualities of the creatures reported on Rorschach Card VIII. Here we have primitive instinctual creatures (salamanders) engaged in sadistic activity, and the whole context was below the level of consciousness (underwater scene).

To summarize, the projective findings were largely a reflection of his perfectionistic, obsessive-compulsive façade. No welter of dynamic materials or symbolic projections appeared. This may be an important theoretical finding in itself. The drawing series did not show body image distortions. His human figures were rigid and tightly compressed laterally, while the male figure and the tree were extended vertically, showing an unusual elongation. The animal drawn was a horse, which was compressed to the bottom of the page so that part of the legs and hoofs extended beyond the lower margin. This showed the need to compress and keep down the instinctual side. His drawings had a bleak starkness about them (even communicated in the upthrusting pine tree), suggestive of some undefinable stigmata, but certainly showing the extreme of isolation and loneliness. Obsessive-compulsive drive was apparent in the detailing of the individual drawings. A specially devised word-association list (125 words) was given the subject, and increased reaction time appeared with most of the emotionally laden items pertinent to his condition. The associations did not add materially to specific insights into his condition. The longest reaction time appeared for the word "dream," and his association was "curse." His sentence completions were virtually a running commentary about his defenses and facade, and reflected an obsessive concern with control, rigidity and the outward face he wished to show to the world. The recall Bender contained no design contaminations and was a virtual duplicate of his perfectionistic original set of designs. The circle of Design A, sometimes regarded as a feminine symbol, was much erased, and the final product was elongated in the vertical axis, giving the impression of bulging strain. A marked emotional disruption appeared when he was asked to write three things which he considered to be impossible. The content of what he wrote was banal, but he indicated that his almost panic-like reaction resulted from feeling that it would be impossible for him to be cured of his "curse." This pattern of divorcing inner experience from performance was typical of the urgency with which the subject always identified with his defense pattern or facade. When urged, he could tell the examiner his feelings, but he would not express them in writing.

DISCUSSION

The Rorschach responses suggested that the subject's masculine development was as minimal as his passivity loomed large. That primitive aggression emerged in his instinctual or impulse life should not obscure the extent to which passive qualities determined the substructure. Little differentiated instinctual vitality had developed, and the wish to nourish this lack may somehow have become connected with the need for blood. That he masturbated with the flow of blood emphasized its relation to his sense of masculine self-esteem. On the other hand, a connection with menstrual blood should not be overlooked, especially since the obsession came about during puberty in an undifferentiated individual. Simultaneous ejaculation with the flow of blood may symbolize denial of castration. The writer is inclined to think of the sexual aspect of the situation as largely a matter of biological puberty having been imposed on what one may most literally call primitive oral fixation. The subject was not equipped for adolescence, much less adult sexual participation. Yet within the sometimes primitive Rorschach matrix he showed at least some degree of development outside the intellect (adaptive use of shading), which would subsume feelings about the needs and desires of others. Apparently, under stress, his adaptive potential and his primitive needs became split apart. Under normal conditions, his strict concern with correct form and perfectionistic standards, together with his considerable intellectual assets, aided him in maintaining the defense facade.

On a broadly theoretical level, the subject literally acted out the pleasure-pain principle. In the midst of self-inflicted wounds which released his very life's blood, he sought pleasure from masturbation. This was tantamount to affirmation of the life principle while he was simultaneously flirting with death. That he flagrantly tampered with paramount taboos of his society was not unlike the vampire, who feeds on existing taboos.

It may be no accident that two of the subject's projections may be linked with Coleridge's *Rime of the Ancient Mariner.* The whole point of the poem was the split between the forces of good and evil. A similar preoccupation virtually ordered the life pattern of the subject. He was himself split between the urge to express his primitive, subhuman needs with others, and the wish to deny them altogether and identify with anything that would testify to uprightness and morality. He chose "an albatross" for the animal he would most like to be. In Coleridge's poem, this bird was the only living creature within the icy barrenness of the polar regions, a pious bird of good omen, who looked to the desolate sailors as if it had a "Christian soul." Instead of a night bird on its primitive, predatory errand, the subject settled for the wish for the white bird of good hope. The ancient mariner, overcome by some inner force of evil, shot the albatross with his crossbow. The sailors hung it around his *neck*, "instead of a cross." The ancient mariner was then caught under a curse or evil spell, until his human compassion overcame his insolent, egocentric identification with the forces of evil and destruction. When this occurred, the albatross fell from his neck into the sea. Hence the saying, "albatross around your neck." The subject most certainly carried a curse around his own neck; his neck had become his *bête noir.* He, like the ancient mariner, was caught in a kind of "life-in-death" vise which would not let go. After destroying the forces of good (albatross) and accepting the forces of evil, the ancient mariner spoke words not dissimilar to the plight of the subject of this study:

> "Fear at my heart, as at a cup
> My life-blood seem'd to sip."

Notice that his response to Rorschach Card IV had to do with undifferentiated sea life (kelp), perhaps a symbol of his unformed masculine side, and a peculiarly original image of "northern lights" for the area of the blot not infrequently associated with the feminine (vagina). Polar lights and the sea continue the atmosphere of Coleridge's poem. Coldness, dark wetness, absence of longed-for color (feeling) and the presence of primitive, primal forces of nature separated the subject from both identification and development along the masculine-feminine scale.

The contrast between the content of the subject's imagery in the performance of the Rorschach and in testing the limits continued the evidence for the split within the subject between good and evil, the world of literal response and the world of imagination and the supernatural, and between reality and unreality. In limits testing, he was merely asked to look through the cards again and see if he could find anything that looked like people. He took to this task literally, and reported human beings for almost every card. Witches, angels and ghosts appeared, along with male beings bent down with heavy burdens. The supernatural world appeared when he was pushed a bit from his defense props and facade. His figure for Card VI supplied another image ("ghost of Christmas past") suggestive of the struggle between the forces of good and evil. The association with Charles Dickens' Scrooge may not be without connection to the way he experienced his father and with heavy burdens he had to carry. At the very least, his masculine development had been bent down and hindered by heavy impedimenta.

So far, we have kept in the main to possibilities associated with the projective findings. Perhaps we have made some progress in understanding something of the structure of the personality involved, but can we call on other kinds of clues to aid in understanding the baffling riddle? We can certainly speculate within the broader frame of knowledge offered by the myth. As a clinical entity, we have no knowledge about this kind of condition, nor any directly comparative materials. Its very existence emphasizes how little is known about the darker recesses of the psyche. That such dark images exist within us cannot be ignored, since behavior has emerged which had hitherto been thought to exist only in folk tale or myth. Because myth itself plays so central a role, we must turn to myth as a source for clarification. The empirical findings of Jung's depth psychology offers a framework for the exploration. It would seem that some long forgotten archetype somehow got dislodged from the murky bottom of the past and emerged to take possession of a modern individual.

From the standpoint of depth psychology, the unconscious may be symbolized by the sea, the great unknown waters, the source from which we came, the boundless repository of nourishment, forces of destruction, and various unknown quanta of virtually inexhaustible extent. Throughout the brief span of man in time, its waters have deposited a plethora of its contents on the shore of a dimly developing consciousness in the form of symbols. These projections from the sea depths became the building blocks for conscious development, and just as evolution has developed within us a physiological isotonic sea-blood essential for life on dry land, the psyche contains the symbol projections necessary for conscious development, archetypal images, a substratum or precursor to consciousness common to all men. This body of symbolic images, now pressed to the bottom of the psyche, combines an infinite number of primordial counterparts which went into the wresting of consciousness as we know it today from the dark past or lack of consciousness. These images are not available to the awarenesses of waking life, but they may be washed up in our dreams. Jung has distinguished between the products of the personal experiences of the individual and those common to all men in the content of dreams. The former is a product of later stages in evolution, while the latter (less close to consciousness) are products of a much earlier stage. He has not attempted to explain the mechanism by which this has occurred, but to describe and interpret what may be empirically observed in dreams. It may be understood, then, that the unconscious can thus be viewed as our symbolical source, the great mother, the feminine principle. Consciousness, its opposite, has been wrested from the unknown into the known, by a constant upward thrust into the light, the masculine principle, that which seeks enlightenment. These two opposing principles, which owe to each other their existence and are renewed in each other, have little to do with a narrow designation of gender or sexual differences as the terms are commonly used. The narrower sexual designations, however, are more concrete end products of the greater macrocosm. This overview may be helpful for some of the subsequent discussion.

It has been indicated that projections of a vampire image are at least as old as the recorded knowledge of man, and that its image has not been confined to any one cultural tradition. This suggests that it must be an archaic image indeed, yet one which has been contained in the psychic substance of man since the dawn of history. Is it merely fascination with the macabre which has insured its survival and kept its form virtually intact? Does its sheer atavism and destructively negative nature justify its survival? Can one simply say that the perverse nature of man would conjure up a vampire image at any stage so as to define evil or contrast it with the good? Perhaps so, but there are many vehicles for so doing, and they are often culture-specific, whereas the vampire image has a strangely universal quality. Is it not reasonable then to assume that the image may have more import than its face value, and that its meaning and universal persistence suggest roots which penetrate deeply into the development of our psychic substance?

Earliest mythology has associated the vampire with the destructive side of the feminine. There can be no doubt but that something destructive was at work within this subject's psyche, and that it took the form of one of the earliest images recorded by man suggests that its history may add to understanding the subject. The negative side of the "great mother" or feminine principle (symbolic of the unconscious itself) has been recognized since earliest times in cultures of the East. This side has been largely ignored by the West, where the feminine principle has been generally assumed to approximate the qualities associated with the Virgin Mary. Neumann (8) has devoted an entire book to the origins of the feminine principle. He has illustrated numerous examples of the positive and negative sides of the feminine in the cults of many cultures. Typical examples include the cults of Kali in India, Hecate in Greece, Osiris in Egypt. Artemis Orthia, the powerful goddess of ancient Sparta, was known as the winged lady, ruler of the kingdom of the beasts. She, as well as Hecate, was not without highly negative traits comparable to vampirism. An ivory plaque survives from the eighth century B.C. (8, p. 274), showing her strangling two large white birds by the neck. Mutilated beasts, from which "a member was cut off," were sacrificed to her. As ruler of primordial mysteries of the feminine, her role was intimately bound up with a sacrifice of blood, or she may have had the power to transform blood into milk. Neumann (8, p. 279) has pointed out that the decisive moments in the life of the female involve blood sacrifice, since they include menstruation, deflowering, conception and childbearing. She (the great mother principle) has both destructive and creative sides, and may demand sacrifice or offer healing and protection, and promote growth. It is her negative side (often vampiristic) that takes many forms and may demand the bloody sacrifice of castration. As female, and as vampire, her (meaning the negative side of the great mother principle) first known image has already been referred to (image on prehistoric Assyrian bowl) earlier in this paper. There are parallels between some of the qualities ascribed to her and some of the behavioral effects apparent in the present subject. What has happened to him seems not dissimilar to demands required by the negative side of Artemis-Hecate when their destructive forces demanded sacrifice. Some mysterious force from the unconscious had sucked away a large part of the life principle in him. It will be remembered that he described both feelings of being loved and feelings of being attacked during his ritual. This would seem similar to having been caught up in the twin forces (positive and negative) which have been ascribed to the power of the feminine principle.

Neumann (7, p. 88) called attention to the youth not strong enough or developed enough to resist the forces symbolized by the overpowering mother, and that his behavior may express flight from incestual fears. He stated that the primary expression of the symbolic "flight" in one under the dominance of the destructive forces of the feminine is self-castration. This, of course, is tantamount to capitulation. The frightening aspect of the powerful mother becomes repressed, but the price required is a ban on sexuality. The son-victim may turn to masturbation or self-castration, but the very idea of coitus or any connection with the female will activate the fear of castration. We know that this subject appears to have acted according to such a sexual ban. Perhaps, then, the vampirism which had him in its clutches hid (or symbolized) the real focus of the fear underlying it, the negative, destructive mother complex. A hostile animal replaced the image of the hostile side of the mother, and the subject virtually acted out the contents of what had been repressed, which is to say, he had taken on the role of the negative aspect of the terrible mother (whose archetype had sucked him in), and like Hecate, he sucked blood from young boys. Since that was one of Hecate's functions when negatively aroused, he may be said to have been under the curse of Hecate, or had developed a "Hecate complex." The Portuguese word for vampire, "bruxsa," contains a similar image, since it refers to a bird-woman who sucks the blood of children (10, p. 522).

The vampire image certainly contains the symbol of the split between the animal nature and the social nature of man. There is the wish to seek life and humanity vicariously, using the means of the wild beast. Stevenson has expressed this dichotomy rather vividly in *Dr. Jekyll and Mr. Hyde*. This patient had been literally caught up in a similar fate.

Using Neumann's (7, pp. 320–329) observations about what happens when archetypes or primitive images become fragmented within the psyche, perhaps we may formulate what may have happened to this subject along similar lines. There had been a riveting of attention upon an unconscious content (archetype of vampirism) in which the libido was sucked away from consciousness onto the archetype. From then on it dominated, which is to say there was no conscious participation with the emergence of the content of the image, while its forces ruled or ordered the life of the victim. The subject became a passive carrier of the projection from the unconscious, and the personality stood in no kind of relationship to what was projected upon it. It became a prisoner. An albatross had been affixed to his neck. When something so archaic as the energy constellated around a vampiristic image had taken hold, and the effects on the individual may amount to having had outer awarenesses and interests sucked away, the individual may very well have come to be experienced by others as set apart or having a stigma, like the witch marks of the Middle Ages. This kind of passive hypnosis by the forces of the unconscious may be present in shamanism and the aura surrounding the witch doctors of primitive cultures.

The foregoing should not be viewed as an explanation of this hitherto unknown form of symptomatology. It has been an attempt to provide a framework from which to view the disorder, and to offer leads about possible origins and process. Its existence makes clear how little is known about psychic forces, once one wanders from the narrow path which winds along familiar ground. What lies in the forest beyond is shrouded in mist, and as yet we have but clumsy means to explore it.

How different the content of the projective findings was from what one might have anticipated. There was nothing bizarre in the sense of autistic material, no turmoil of sexual symbols or reversals, and none of the flood of psychotic thought that could naturally have been expected. Instead, there was a repetition of obsessive-compulsive facade, profound depression, degrees of raw primitiveness, and an over-alert obsession to avoid participation with what may have been psychopathic-sadistic pressure. He must be schizophrenic, one thinks. Perhaps he may become so, but no extensive evidence appeared to support it as an on-going process at that time. There were no psychotic fragments in his handwriting and the drawings were not psychotic. Does this mean that the projective stimuli simply failed to ferret out the underlying psychosis? Perhaps, but the Rorschach commonly elicits a flood of psychotic intrusions in any number of psychotic patients. Why not here? The only plausible answer seems to lie in the assumption that the material was not there or that there was something different in the psychic makeup of the subject. We have wandered from the path of the known, and known explanations may not account for anything but the surface features in this complex subject.

Over a period of time, the writer has had the opportunity to examine and report on some unique conditions. These conditions were widely diverse, but carried the common bond of cases of individuals having had *in vivo* experiences of phenomena ordinarily expected to be symbolic or, as in this case, non-existent. The interesting thing about them is that they all appeared to be remarkably stable in relation to the extent of trauma with which they had to cope. One of these involved a true hermaphrodite (4), who was investigated via projective techniques just before and directly following two sets of operations separated by months of time (breast and genital), and the subject was followed over a period of more than a year. There was no upheaval of unconscious materials during these emotionally charged circumstances. It was not just that the subject was an hermaphrodite, but anatomical changes were being made. Others have reported that hermaphrodites tended to be stable, but none have been studied under the conditions described above. In an investigation (5) of the fantasies of children who knew they were soon to die, a study (9) of Icelandic children whose bodies were battered and scarred through having had extremely high thresholds for pain, and a study (6) of a transsexualite who had partially changed her sexual characteristics (mastectomy) and was determined to remove the rest of her female sexual features, there was found a relative lack of overall unconscious disruptions or evidence for impending psychosis. This is not to say that the subjects of those studies were not disturbed, but that they were not disturbed to the extent one might legitimately expect. To a considerable extent, the same was true of the subject of the present investigation. Some six years ago, the writer examined another true hermaphrodite, an adolescent, who did show some degree of psychotic thinking. Recently, this same adolescent was examined in another setting and was again thought to have had borderline psychotic qualities. Yet, many areas were intact both previously and now. The psychotic features may have been irrelevant to the fact that he was an hermaphrodite, but he showed some surprising strengths despite both.

Perhaps there is a liminal range for psychosis. Perhaps there is only a certain range of internal and external events in combination that will produce what we call psychosis. If this is true, we will have to extend our narrow concept of the continuum of psychic disorders to include a state hitherto not recognized, a kind of psychic limbo, which enables some individuals to adjust to internal conditions we often assume may produce psychosis. Perhaps, when symbol becomes fact, there is nothing to project. We have as yet to learn the nature of the effects the emergence of archaic material has on the nature of the defenses. It may have been that in this subject, nothing archaic remained unconscious, symbol became fact. This may have been why the defenses, at least in relation to society, appeared relatively intact. If subjects who can be assumed to experience the ultimate in actual trauma can somehow find an oasis of rest within themselves, or can climb onto a relatively stable plateau, then cannot we expect the same potential to exist in overt psychosis? It may be that psychosis is simply unrelated by cause and effect to these phenomena. A handful of peculiar cases offers a poor medium for generalizations. We simply may not have seen enough of such cases, and if we had, we might find the same statistical relationship to the occurrence of psychosis as found in the population at large. Yet it may be that in just these kinds of cases that we will find important checks which can be applied to current theoretical assumptions. At the very least, the present study suggests that a personality can be reasonably well organized quite aside from a core of highly primitive needs which had been acted out.

In a final word on vampirism, perhaps it can be said that the image is not so wholly negative as it appears. It has been suggested that it may serve as a vehicle for the expression of the most negative side of the larger view of the feminine principle. By feminine principle, we have not meant the individual mother of the subject, but the feminine side of life development; more, that the unconscious itself may be symbolized by it. This subject seemed to have been obsessed in such a way that forced him to tamper with the life force and experiment with the death force. His remarks about color symbolism on Rorschach Card II offered this possible interpretation from his own association. On the one hand, the vampire symbolizes the ever-constant wish for life and renewal (a positive component), while on the other hand, it is the symbol of the hideously egocentric wish for survival that would destroy a living human being so as to maintain its own existence (a destructive component). If one views death as equivalent to the unconscious, and life as equivalent to the coursing of warm blood, the vampire can be seen as the projection of the image of the struggle for life. In one of the most sacred religious rituals of our own culture, the Holy Communion, we drink red wine-blood to renew ourselves, and to symbolize the triumph of the forces of life over death. In this patient, however, the primitive desire appeared to have become an end in itself. Perhaps its parasitic nature reflected the paradox of one principle existing at the expense of its opposite, a death battle, in which the unconscious fed on, and sapped the life away from consciousness. For the patient, the destructive, negative forces dominated, yet somewhere within him, something searched for an albatross alive again, and pointed the way to hope. This may suggest that even at our worst, we are not entirely without some contact with our best, if we can learn to recognize it.

SUMMARY

The projective findings in a case of auto-vampirism were presented and an interpretation was offered to provide a basis for understanding the personality structure of the patient. The historical development of the vampire image in myth was reviewed and used to throw light on its possible significance and to offer clues as to how it may have appeared in the subject. The emergence of a vampiristic pattern was analyzed within the framework of depth psychology, and its implications for theoretical processes were discussed.

REFERENCES

1. Campbell, J. Commentary. In *Grimm's Fairy Tales*. Pantheon, New York, 1956.
2. Fenichel, O. *The Psychoanalytic Theory of Neurosis*. Norton, New York, 1945.
3. Jones, E. *On the Nightmare*. Hogarth Press, London, 1931.
4. McCully, R. S. A projective study of a true hermaphrodite during a period of radical surgical procedures. Psychiat. Quart. [Suppl.], 32: 1–36, 1958.
5. McCully, R. S. Fantasy productions of children with a progressively crippling and fatal illness. J. Genet. Psychol., 102: 203–213, 1963.
6. McCully, R. S. An interpretation of projective findings in a case of female transsexualism. J. Project. Techn., 27: 436–446, 1963.
7. Neumann, E. *The Origins and History of Consciousness*. Pantheon, New York, 1954.
8. Neumann, E. *The Great Mother*. Pantheon, New York, 1955.
9. Pétursson, E., Tryggvason, G. and McCully, R. S. Infantile ("congenital") indifference

to pain: A clinical study of an Icelandic family in which three brothers showed the characteristic syndrome. In *Proceedings of Third World Congress of Psychiatry, Vol. I*, pp. 495–500. Univ. of Toronto Press, Toronto, and McGill Univ. Press, Montreal, 1962.

10. Robbins, R. H. *The Encyclopedia of Witchcraft and Demonology.* Crown, New York, 1959.
11. Summers, M. *The Vampire.* University Books, New York, 1960.

3

Cannibalism and Vampirism in Paranoid Schizophrenia

M. BENEZECH, *M.D.*[1]
M. BOURGEOIS, *M.D.*[2]
D. BOUKHABZA, *M.D.*[3]
J. YESAVAGE, *M.D.*[4]

This study reports an unusual case of cannibalism and vampirism in a paranoid schizophrenic. Such cases are rare in developed countries[1,2] but the basic drives which led to this act are common. This case should be of particular interest since there were many indications that this patient would eventually commit a violent act, which were ignored by the authorities.

[1,2]Unité d'Enseignment et Récherche, University of Bordeaux II, France.
[3,4]VA Medical Center. Palo Alto, California: Department of Psychiatry and Behavioral Sciences. Stanford University School of Medicine, Stanford, California.

THE CASE

The subject was born in 1940 into a family of devout Catholics in a rural area of France, the Mayenne, where witchcraft is still practiced. There was extensive psychiatric illness in the family with his father taking early retirement for depressive illness, another sister with depression and a schizophrenic brother. The patient's childhood was unremarkable except for his family's strict discipline.

The patient had his first psychiatric evaluation in 1958 at age 18 for "emotional outbursts" but was not diagnosed schizophrenic or hospitalized. In 1965 he married a paranoid schizophrenic with whom he had two children. His first overt psychotic episode occurred in 1969 when he suddenly decided to attempt to strangle a neighbor with his wife's help. He was not convicted for lack of evidence. When hospitalized for a medical condition in 1971 he was diagnosed schizophrenic for the first time. By 1975 he was floridly psychotic and made several journeys across Europe on religious missions at the request of God.

The series of events which led to his arrest began in 1978 when he attempted to strangle another neighbor. The subject was not arrested despite the complaints of the neighbor. Later that year his wife died of an apparent drowning. In September 1979 the subject went on a rampage which started with an attempted rape and vampire attack on a 9 year old girl. This episode was thwarted by the lucky appearance of the child's mother but the subject escaped. On the same evening, he attacked and killed with a stick a 60 year-old man and devoured large pieces of the victim's thigh and tried to suck his blood from the femoral artery. The following day he broke into a farm but was surprised by the owners and forced to leave, however, he later returned and beat unconscious the farmer and his maid. The farmer's wife tried to defend herself with a pitchfork but the subject disarmed her and killed her and her husband with it. The maid survived with spinal cord injuries having been left for dead. The subject finally was arrested on his way home and later admitted that he had in fact murdered his wife and disguised the act as a drowning.

The subject was tried and found not guilty by reason of insanity and transferred to Cadillac Hospital Security Department where he has been under evaluation by the first two authors. During all evaluations the subject never seemed to understand the seriousness of his situation even after treatment with neuroleptics. The patient was oriented and was calm, relaxed and smiling, without reticence or feelings of guilt. The mood was often elevated with inappropriate smiles. The delusions which started in 1975 governed his life and were present during the examination. These were associated with auditory hallucinations. No other Schneiderian criteria were present. He explained his wife's murder saying that she was willing to die and take him with her in death so he decided to kill her first to circumvent her intentions. About the multiple murders in September 1979 he stated that God's voice told him to kill everybody. He depicts the first killing of that day in a completely delusional way: he wanted to prove that he was bad and then ate the body to recover God: "I ate his flesh and drank his blood to obey the sentence: Who will eat my body and drink my blood will live."* The patient's intellectual level was normal as were all physical, laboratory and electroencephalographic evaluations.

DISCUSSION

In psychoanalytic theory, "cannibalism" related to the sado-oral stage when, after the sucking stage, the child feels the need to bite.[3] The basic ambivalence and conflict between biting and being bitten is resolved with the development of a "cannibalistic taboo." Similar taboos against murder and incest are developed respectively at the anal and phallic stages. Despite its taboo nature in the developed world, cannibalism is seen in some primitive societies with group participation aiming at incorporating the victim or enemy's qualities.[4,5] This perspective was not lost to Freud who argued that primitive herd brothers killed and devoured the father to appropriate his power.[6] Finally, cannibalism and vampirism are present in language, in the form of verbal metaphors (to devour someone with one's eyes), as well as in literature and myths.[7,8] Thus it seems that the idea of cannibalism may be more basic to our lives than one might want to believe.

Although cases such as this are rare, they emphasize certain clinical points. First, though the incidence of crimes committed by schizophrenics may or may not equal that of the general population, schizophrenics do in fact commit serious crimes. A recent study completed by the authors suggests that paranoid schizophrenics are particularly

*Note: The scriptural basis for this is probably John: 6:54. This statement is also clarified at 6:63 where the point is made that the religious benefit spiritually not corporally from communion.

likely to commit crimes involving injury to others.[9] This study also found that such patients like the one in this case often attack people they know. Finally, it should be noted that this subject gave ample warning, ignored by the authorities, by assaulting two people before his four murders.

REFERENCES

1. Burton-Bradley, BG: Cannibalism for cargo. J Nerv Ment Dis 163: 428–431. 1976.
2. Vandenbergh RL and Kelly JF: Vampirism. Arch Gen. Psychiatry 11: 543–547. 1964.
3. Fenichel O: the Psychoanalytic Theory of Neuroses. New York. Norton. 1945.
4. Harris M: Cannibales et Monarques Essai sur L'origine des Cultures. Paris. Flammarion. 1979.
5. Staden H: Nus. Feroces et Anthropophages. Paris. Metailie. 1979.
6. Freud S: Totem and Taboo: New York. Random House. 1960.
7. Penrose V: La Comtesse Sanglante. Paris. Mercure de France. 1969.
8. Vadim R: Histoires de Vampires. Paris. Laffont. 1961.
9. Benezech M. Bourgeois M and Yesavage J: Violence in the mentally ill: A study of 547 patients in a French hospital for the criminally insane. J Nerv Ment Dis. 1980.

4

Clinical Vampirism

A Presentation of 3 Cases and a Reevaluation of Haigh, the "Acid-Bath Murderer"

R. E. HEMPHILL,
M.A., M.D., D.P.M., F.R.C. Psych.[1]
T. ZABOW,
M.B., Ch.B., F.F. Psych., (S.A.), D.P.M.[2]

SUMMARY

Clinical vampirism is named after the mythical vampire, and is a recognizable, although rare, clinical entity characterized by periodic compulsive blood-drinking, affinity with the dead and uncertain identity. It is hypothetically the expression of an inherited archaic myth, the act of taking blood being a ritual that gives temporary relief. From ancient times vampirists have given substance to belief in the existence of supernatural vampires.

Four vampirists, including Haigh, the "acid-bath mur-

[1] [2]Department of Psychiatry, University of Cape Town, South Africa

Reprinted with permission from *South African Medical Journal*, 1983, Vol. 63, 278–281.

derer," are described. From childhood they cut themselves, drank their own, exogenous human or animal blood to relieve a craving, dreamed of bloodshed, associated with the dead, and had a changing identity. They were intelligent, with no family mental or social pathology.

Some self-cutters are auto-vampirists; females are not likely to assault others for blood, but males are potentially dangerous. Vampirism may be a cause of unpredictable repeated assault and murder, and should be looked for in violent criminals who are self-mutilators. No specific treatment is known.

Vampirism has been reported in the medical literature for more than a century. It was named after the mythical vampire in order to describe the sucking of blood or drinking of blood to satisfy a craving for it. An interest in the dead has also been recorded, so that vampirism has been confused with necrophilia.

Single cases and an extensive bibliography have been published by Kayton,[1] McCully [2] and Bourguignon.[3] Their term 'auto-vampirism' is convenient but misleading, for subjects may take their own and/or exogenous blood. Of the latest definitions: '(*a*) belief in vampires, (*b*) acts and practices of vampires, blood sucking, (*c*) necrophilism',[4] only (*b*) is appropriate, and the concept requires clarification.

The essential characteristic of the vampire was that he drank fresh blood specifically to satisfy a need, also having an abnormal interest in death and the dead. The appropriate clinical substantive for a human who displays these characteristics is "vampirist," not vampire, which refers to a supernatural creature or to a bat.

The mythical vampire was an evil spirit which, being refused entry into the "other world" because of unsuitable behaviour in life or neglect of rituals, returned to the grave as a "revenant" or "living dead" being. He re-animated his corpse and sustained it with blood sucked from the living during sleep, or by biting the neck and drinking from the wound. A victim thus attacked or a suicide victim was liable to become a vampire. Vampires lived in cemeteries and seldom left their graves except to satisfy their need for blood: the dead were their people.[5] The vampire did not desecrate graves, violate corpses, eat human flesh or have sexual intercourse with the living. He had no real identity and was thought not to cast a shadow or reflect an image in a mirror.[1] The characteristics of a periodic craving for blood, association with the dead and no certain identify are a triad also found in clinical vampirism.

The vampire myth is of great antiquity and appears in some form in most religions that hold a belief in a corporate existence for the spirit after death. It entered Europe from Asia Minor and moved west through Romania and Hungary. The word vampire, of Turkish or Magyar origin, was first used in English in 1734.[2] The vampire has featured in German, French, English and American romantic and horrific literature since the late 18th century, and novels, plays and films derived from *Dracula*[6] continue to proliferate. There is a substratum of fact to Dracula and the associated Frankenstein, based on historical persons.[7,8]

The drinking of blood may be a feature of sadomasochism, blood rituals, fetishism, ritual revenge, psychosis, and drug intoxication.[9] Most of the striking cases collected by Krafft-Ebing[10] appear not to have been vampirists. Vampirism is not a primary symptom of any other psychiatric or psychopathic disorder, and its specific motive distinguishes it from other blood-related aberrations. The condition is not likely to be discovered except in criminal cases where evidence is restricted by judicial rulings, and by chance via psychiatric examinations or surgical treatment of self-injuries. Some of our patients who carry out self-mutilation cut themselves in order to suck blood. They had an impaired sense of identity; 2 could not recognize their faces in the mirror and some expressed an interest in death. The mirror effect indicates a gross disturbance of personal reality and is sometimes found in schizophrenia and unreality states as well as vampirism.[1] Identity is the innate knowledge of individuality which becomes more certain and firm as the child develops.

We suggest that compulsive blood-taking, uncertain identity and an abnormal interest in death, as observed in our cases and reported variously by others, are symptoms of the psychopathology of clinical vampirism. Uncertain identity is probably invariable, while an interest in death may not always be evident.

In addition to non-criminal vampirists, we have intensively studied 3 who had been charged with dishonesty and referred for psychiatric assessment because of self-mutilation. We have also re-examined the case of Haigh, "acid-bath" murderer of 1949, regarding whom there was much inconclusive controversy in psychiatric circles, and propose that he was also a vampirist. We describe these 4 cases in detail, refer to others and discuss clinical vampirism and its implications.

In this article vampirism may refer to the clinical condition or to the practice of "drinking" or "sucking" blood, according to the context.

CASE REPORTS

John Haigh

John Haigh, the "acid-bath" murderer, was executed in London on 10 August 1949 at the age of 40. Haigh confessed that between September 1944 and February 1949 he had killed 9 persons, incised their necks and drunk a cupful of blood from each. Six were friends whose property he then acquired by fraud, but the other 3 were unidentified casual strangers. The primary motive for all the murders, he said, was an irresistible urge for blood, and not gain: 'there are so many other ways of making easy money, though illegitimately'.[11] Lord Dunboyne[11] wrote: 'No other reported case traceable seems to suggest that a murderer drank the blood of the murdered as an end in itself, unassociated with any sexual perversion'.

A wealth of material exists, giving quite a good picture of his first 25 and last 5 years, but there is little regarding the intervening period of prison sentences and the war. The following is derived from a book on the trial of Haigh, edited by Lord Dunboyne,[11] and a biography by La Bern,[12] the two of which complement each other.

Haigh was the only child of sound, middle-class parents for whom he showed genuine affection throughout life. His birth, development and health were normal, there were no congenital or blood disorders, and no family history of mental instability. Intelligent and musical, he was a schoolboy organist and chorister at Wakefield Cathedral, and had a good character. However, between the ages of 25 and 34 he served three prison sentences for dishonesty and company swindles, forgery and impersonation. Thereafter he had business interests in London and lived in the Onslow Court residential hotel. He had close, well-to-do, respectable friends who never suspected that he was a criminal; they corresponded with him even after he was convicted. He was arrested and charged with the murder of Mrs. Deacon, a 69-year-old widow who lived in the Onslow Court Hotel, in February 1949.

Apart from crime, his adult behaviour was unremarkable both in and out of prison. From childhood he was good-natured, fastidious and generous. He loved animals and children and disliked cruelty and violence. When his wife left him a few months after their marriage at the age of 25 he had no further interest in sex. He lived well, drank moderately, did not take drugs and did not associate with criminals outside of prison.

He was not impulsive and showed caution in his frauds, in contrast to the recklessness of his murders.

He enjoyed blood, and from the age of 6 would lick scratches and wound himself to suck it. He pictured and dreamed of people injured and bleeding after railway accidents. Although of the Plymouth Brethren, he was fascinated by Holy Communion and the Crucifixion, and sometimes saw blood pouring from a large crucifix that hung over the altar in the cathedral, while the bleeding figure of Christ would appear in his dreams.

In 1944, when he was 35, blood dripped into his mouth from an accidental scalp wound. That night he dreamed that his "mouth was full of blood, which revived the old taste," and knew that he would have to obtain blood. He killed 2 persons that year, 3 in 1945, 3 in 1948 and Mrs. Deacon in February 1949. He said, "Before each of my killings I had a series of dreams, I saw a forest of crucifixes that changed into green trees dripping with blood . . . which I drank, and once more I awakened with a desire that demanded fulfilment" . . . "The dream cycles started early in the week and culminated on Friday"(i.e. the day of the Crucifixion—author's note).

In anticipation of having to kill he arranged to have the use of the storeroom of a small factory in Crawley, where he installed noncorrosive metal drums, carboys of sulphuric acid, a pump, tools, and protective clothing. He would club or shoot the victim in the head, plug the wound, incise the neck, draw a cupful of blood and "drink it for 3 to 5 minutes, after which I felt better." He would put the body in the drum and pump acid over it. The process of dissolution took a few days and he visited the workshop daily to inspect. If the body had to be dismembered he greased the floor first, so that the blood would not sink in and he could wash it away. The "sludge" was poured down the drain and the drum, with what did not dissolve, such as plastic articles or dentures, was thrown on the rubbish heap of the factory yard.

He drove Mrs. Deacon to see an "invention" at his workshop, shot her and drank her blood. She weighed 200 lb. and, exhausted after getting the body into the barrel, he went to Crawley for tea. He then completed his task, dined and drove back to London. He openly sold Mrs. Deacon's jewellery to a shop and sent her bloodstained coat to a cleaner, all of which was easily traced. The police found blood and other incriminating evidence at the workshop. Haigh confessed and voluntarily described the other 8 murders, then unknown to the police. He told his last visitor before his execution the "real truth"—"I was impelled to kill by wild blood demons, the spirit inside me commanded me to kill."

Haigh seemed not to realize that he might die or that the disintegrating bodies had once been alive and his friends. His only regret was that "being led by an irresistible urge, I was not given to the discovery of the distress this might cause to myself and others," by which he meant his parents and friends. He wrote to his mother from the death cell: "My spirit will remain earthbound for a while. My mission is not yet fulfilled." Haigh was unconcerned about his trial and refused to appeal against his sentence. A panel of psychiatrists found that he was not legally insane and that he had no symptoms of mental illness; his electro-encephalogram (EEG) was normal.

On the grounds that his impeccable early career, usually good character and personal fastidiousness could not be reconciled with the gruesome killings, it was suggested that Haigh had a multiple personality or identity. A non-violent, cautious, professional swindler is unlikely to murder for money and to do so recklessly. Haigh kept the same friends during his last 5 years, stayed in their houses and escorted their teenage daughters to entertainments. None suspected anything sinister of him. There seems no doubt that Haigh's identity, and the motives and values that corresponded with it, were not constant. Haigh realized this when, normally self-assured, he said: "No-one will ever understand me, I am really very bewildering."

The three unmarried White males described below all came from good middle-class homes with stable, affectionate parents and siblings, and no family psychopathology. Birth and development were normal, and they were well-built, reasonably good-looking and, apart from self-mutilation, physically and mentally healthy and free from congenital defects or blood disorders. In all the central nervous system and EEGs were normal, and their IQs 110–120. All found cannibalism revolting and films about Dracula "rubbish." They were not interested in the occult or religion, and had no food fads.

Personal Case 1

This 27-year-old had been expelled from 5 schools between the ages of 8 and 13 and thereafter detained in residential schools, reformatories, prisons and a treatment unit, except when he absconded and when released for 7 months at the age of 20 and 3 months at the age of 26. His offences included drug trafficking, housebreaking, stealing, fraud, impersonation and assaults (some unprovoked) in prison and outside. He never earned a remission of sentence and was eventually declared a habitual criminal. He took pot (marijuana), speed (a mixture of cocaine, heroin and morphine), LSD, cocaine and other drugs until the age of 20, after which he took only dagga and drank alcohol.

He was an attractive, willful child, liable to tantrums, violence and cruelty. From the age of 4 he burned curtains, smashed furniture, bashed his teddy bear against the wall, mutilated his pet birds and chameleons, hanged his dog and cat and terrorized the school.

He was always impulsive, reckless, vindictive and incapable of remorse. Violence, human injuries and blood excited him, but he got no pleasure out of inflicting pain. He relieved frustration in prison by tearing rats apart and indulging in the blood. He was a passive homosexual and masochist who enjoyed pain inflicted by others but found accidental pain unpleasant. Corporal punishment excited a "wonderful feeling" with sexual arousal, and sex was satisfying only when he was sodomized violently.

From the age of 4 he sucked his blood and later cut himself and opened veins longitudinally for the purpose. From the age of 24 he had dreams of tying a boy to a tree and slashing him. When the blood spouted in his dreams, he wakened "satisfied and drained." After such dreams a desire for exogenous blood led him to buy fresh blood at the abattoir and drink it with "a warm relaxed feeling, not sexual." He would bite the neck or shoulder of his partners to suck their blood, and sometimes thought of cutting them with a knife. The craving subsided for several weeks after taking his own or exogenous blood. Blood "warmed and relaxed" him; alcohol and drugs did not influence the blood interest.

From childhood he dreamed of being dead and kept dead creatures in his room. At the age of 26 he visited cemeteries in the hope of exhuming a fresh body, and longed to have one to "cherish it." He never had necrophiliac sexual desires. He would visualize himself as dead and "longed to have cancer" like his mother so as to experience her suffering "inside" and her death. He falsely confessed to having murdered a child in the hope of "seeing what it was like to be hanged," as he believed that only one part of him would die and the other would observe execution. His identity was never certain. He had three separate names and separate prison records, "I am never sure which I am at any time," he said.

At 27 he had "blood dreams" and an increasing urge to cut a young homosexual friend for blood, and would have done so eventually if he had not been arrested for suspected car theft.

In hospital he was superficially pleasant, moody and unsociable. He liked to speak of death and blood fantasies, and made sinister drawings in red ink, which might well illustrate the blood demons of Haigh. He sometimes cut himself and sucked blood. After leaving hospital he received a long prison sentence for violence and other serious crimes.

Personal Case 2

This 19-year-old had been sent to a reformatory. From the age of 17 he had travelled around the country associating with criminals, living by crime, and indulging heavily in drugs and alcohol. He was grossly psychopathic but had some feeling for his parents. Since childhood he had been prone to tantrums and violence, and was unfeeling, impulsive, vindictive and incapable of remorse. He tormented animals and children and committed arson.

From the age of 16 he had stabbed strangers on impulse, "some of whom may have died." He enjoyed burning shops, robbing, smashing windows and stealing cards during political riots. Recurrent dreams of violence, blood and mutilated people "gave him peace." He had no real interest in sex and feared he might kill a sexual partner.

As regards blood he said: "I have liked the appearance and taste of blood all my life. I would lick scratches and cut myself for it. I used to pull off birds' heads and drink their blood, I bit the head off a guinea pig when I was a child and sucked the blood, and pulled off the head of a chicken, collected the blood in my hands and drank it. I cut myself in order to get blood. Blood relaxes me. I think if I got it every few days, I would be settled. When I feel annoyed, the sight of blood usually calms me, but if it does not, I smash my fists against the wall and lick the blood, even tear my clothes up. It is the feeling of blood in me not the taste that I need, I would like to get it from another person, but so far have not worked out how."

From about the age of 6 he had kept dead animals in his room and talked to the dead in the graveyard. He still envied them, and asked,

"Are they as unhappy as I am?" He never knew who he really was: "I can't understand myself, so how could other people understand me?" In order to attain an identify he joined the Cape Scorpions, an exclusive criminal gang, and was tattooed with their emblem, but never identified with them.

In hospital he was restless and unpredictable, but not violent. He would cut himself for blood whenever possible, and once managed to lick blood from a used syringe. When prevented from taking a table knife he began to shake, sweat, and shout that he must have blood and would have to smash a window and cut someone with the glass. He then bashed his knuckles against the wall and sucked the blood. After sedation he settled down. We learned later that he died after a surgical operation.

Personal Case 3

This 22-year-old broke his arm at the age of 5, and at the age of 8 smashed his right knee with loss of patella and tissue, in road accidents. He enjoyed hospital and picked off the skin grafts in order both to prolong his stay and suck blood. From the age of 13 he mutilated himself in other ways, was hospitalized many times and, to date, has received many blood transfusions when exsanguinated and more than 200 anaesthetics. From the age of 17 to 21 (between spells in hospital) he worked in offices for short periods. He missed much of his schooling, but educated himself in hospital. From childhood he had been reserved and well-behaved; he objected to pain, cruelty and violence and loved animals. He had no interest in sex, alcohol or drugs. He said: "I have never been upset by the sight of blood, but enjoyed it tremendously. When I was young it was a habit to suck blood, which soon became a craving and I had to have it. I cut myself to get blood, but as I dislike pain, I usually get it by scraping the granulations which does not hurt much, collecting a cupful and drinking it. I get the craving frequently. I cannot say what sets it off. I have always liked the taste of blood, but it is the feeling of having it inside me that is important, and a transfusion is more satisfying than drinking it" . . . "I was always fascinated by death and from the age of 4 visited cemeteries, hoping to see bodies and bones."

He enjoyed surgical and accident wards, seeing the sick and dying, helping nurses with patients' dressings and watching blood transfusions. He asked, unsuccessfully, to work in the mortuary and postmortem rooms. He mutilated himself for blood and to get back into hospital. "Blood, sickness and death are all connected in some ways. I would love to be dead. I would love to have the experience of death. I would really love it. I have no real idea who I am, I am often scared of what, whoever I am, might do." He only felt real in a hospital. For a few weeks after leaving he was free from unreal feelings and the desire for blood. He rapidly became unsettled, injured himself and was urgently admitted to a hospital. While he was under observation in this hospital he was quiet and unsociable. He managed to cut himself or scrape his wound occasionally to suck blood. During the few years since his discharge he has continued to injure himself very severely.

DISCUSSION

These 4 subjects each displayed the triad of vampirism. They ingested their own and exogenous blood from victims (Haigh), partners and abattoirs (case 1), animals and clinical specimens (case 2), and blood transfusions (case 3). They frequently dreamed of bloodshed and death.

Death attracted them, not as a release from suffering but because they wished to "experience it" as "living dead" in the company of the dead. Cases 1–3 frequented cemeteries, talked to the graves, and kept dead creatures. Haigh spent time with his decomposing victims. In one way or another all expressed a belief that in dying they would achieve another, more real existence.

Their identities were changeable and uncertain. Haigh appeared to develop satisfactorily to adulthood; he fluctuated thereafter, and the fastidious, socially acceptable young man cannot be recognized in the callous, revolting murderer. Case 1 had several identifies; cases 2 and 3 had no clear idea of themselves, and found their predicament bewildering.

Their personalities were different. Haigh, non-violent and sociable, murdered 9 people. Case 3, a non-violent and introverted man, inflicted terrible injuries on himself and later attacked others. Cases 1 and 2, violent, impulsive psychopaths, did not assault for blood, although they both contemplated it. Therefore vampirism, although specifically psychopathic, is not necessarily associated with general or violent psychopathic disorder and, conceivably, might occur in persons not recognized as abnormal, for example Haigh.

All had satisfactory family, medical and psychiatric histories. Vampirism and psychopathy developed in spite of favourable influences and no possible causes for either were discovered. The patients were disinterested in sex, and blood evoked no sexual feeling, in contrast with a very rare form of sadomasochism in which drinking a partner's blood is said to cause sexual arousal and orgasm. Alcohol and drugs were not relevant factors.

Mental unrest and an increasing desire for blood preceded each indulgence. Recurrent blood dreams sometimes dramatized the urgency, and Haigh said he would have to kill for blood shortly after a significant dream. The visions of bleeding forests and crucifixes of Haigh and case 1, and the latter's drawing of a blood demon must have had a similar origin in their unconscious.

Taking a taste or a cupful of blood was followed by a warm, relaxed feeling, with calm and disappearance of the craving. This lasted from 1 day to months, perhaps longer. It is not known whether Haigh took his own blood between murders. The indulgence was neither a habit nor an addiction. Vampirism is a rare compulsive disorder with an irresistible urge for blood ingestion, a ritual necessary to bring mental relief; like other compulsions, its meaning is not understood by the participant.

Any theory about vampirism is speculative. What we propose assumes the unconscious persistence of ancient myths. In mythology blood contained the essence and qualities of the host which could be transferred to another. Thus a victor drank the blood of his enemy in order to possess his powers,[13] and a vampire sucked blood from the living in order to obtain regeneration.

Archaic man's fear of a blood-sucking spirit and of becoming a 'revenant' became an archetypal myth from which human vampirism evolved. The human vampirist is analogous to the vampire, with the common features of the main triad and unease, isolation and the "mirror defect." The activities of the human vampirist throughout the ages may have given real substance to the belief in the vampire and reinforced the myth. Vampirism today is therefore a rare atavism and blood-taking a ritual act of regeneration.

How common is vampirism? A few cases of probable vampirism have been published, such as Krafft-Ebing's [10] case No. 31 who paid to prick women and suck their blood. McCully's case who from the age of 13 periodically cut his neck and caught the blood in his mouth, and tried unsuccessfully to involve another boy, and Bourguignon's[3] female patient who repeatedly sucked blood from a pharyngeal angioma, later bleeding to death.

The occurrence of self-mutilation and other assaults on the body appears to have increased in the last 25 years; self-cutters are predominantly female and many have an impaired sense of identity. A few cut themselves primarily to drink blood, and we have found 7—4 females and 3 males—all auto-vampirists, among 150 non-criminal self-mutilators. Taking blood from others seems to be an exclusively male phenomenon. This is probably because force is involved and females seem to have an inbuilt bias against criminal violence; the large majority of convictions for serious assault and murder in Western countries are among males.

Vampirism seems to vary in frequency and intensity, from our fully developed cases to the disturbed young women who occasionally cut themselves to taste their blood. Nothing is known about remission or permanent resolution; there is no specific treatment.

Since vampirism involves unprovoked violence against the subject or another person it might be regarded as a variant of sadomasochism; there is insufficient evidence to show whether this may be the case. In vampirism the specific motive is to obtain and ingest blood, and not indulgence in cruelty, self-punishment or self-degradation, and therefore in our view it is not essentially sadomasochistic and is a clinical entity.

Although rare, vampirism has serious clinical and practical implications. Male auto-vampirists may attack others for blood; both males and females are a recurrent treatment problem. Self-mutilation is not rare among violent recidivist prisoners,[14] some of whom may be vampirists. The circumstances, motives and blood interest of criminals who mutilate themselves, or who have scars from repeated self-mutilation, should be inquired into carefully. Old and recent scars, together with puncture wounds convenient for sucking blood, are very suspicious.

Vampirism is thus a possible cause of unpredictable repeated murder which is likely to be overlooked.

The vampirist may show no obvious signs of mental disorder. It is a disturbing thought that a pleasant person, like Haigh, unsuspected, may be a vampirist liable to a periodic craving for blood.

REFERENCES

1. Kayton NL. The relationship of the vampire legend to schizophrenia. *J Youth Adolesc* 1972; 1: 303–314.
2. McCully RS. Vampirism: historical perspective and underlying process in relation to a case of auto-vampirism. *J Nerv Ment Dis* 1964: 139: 440–452.
3. Bourguignon A. Situation du vampirisme et de l'autovampirisme. *Ann Med Psychol* 1977; 1: 181–196.
4. Osol A, ed. *Blakiston's Gould Medical Dictionary.* 3rd ed. New York: McGraw Hill, 1972: 1631.
5. Robins RH. *Encyclopedia of Witchcraft and Demonology.* New York: Peter Nevill, 1979; 521–525.
6. Stoker B. *Dracula.* New York: Modern Library, 1897.
7. Florescu R., MacNall RT. *In Search of Dracula.* Greenwich, Conn.: New York Graphic Society. 1972.
8. Florescu R., *In Search of Frankenstein.* London: New English Library, 1975.
9. Bugliosi V., with Gentry C. *Helter Skelter: the Manson Murders.* London: Penguin Books, 1975: 102.
10. Krafft-Ebing R. *Psychopathia Sexualis.* New York: GP Putnams, 1965: 99–125.
11. Lord Dunboyne. *The Trial of John George Haigh*, Notable British Trials Series, vol. 78. London: William Hodge, 1953.
12. La Bern A. *Haigh–the Mind of a Murderer.* London: WH Allen, 1974.
13. Tannahill R. *Flesh and Blood–A History of the Cannibal Complex.* London: Hamish Hamilton, 1975: 120–136.
14. Bach-y-Rita G. Habitual violence and self-mutilation. *Am J Psychiatry* 1974: 131: 1010–1020.

5

Vampirism
A Clinical Condition

HERSCHEL PRINS, *M Phil.*[1]

The phenomenon of the vampire is ancient, ubiquitous, and fascinating; moreover, it can only be understood adequately within the context of more general blood reliefs and rituals. (See Prins, 1984 for a review). References to vampires and associated phenomena may be found in the world's great literature long before Bram Stoker created his notorious and evil Count (Summers, 1960, 1980). Belief in the vampire's actual physical existence was probably encouraged by the prevalent practice of premature burial during times of plague, by the large numbers of itinerants and beggars that abound at such times, and by the fact that many of them took refuge in vaults and graveyards. In addition, the myth was probably given more tangible reality by such physical explanations as *Erythropoietic Protoporphyria* or its variants. This disorder is said to induce the body to produce an excess of porphyria, which results not only in excess redness of the eyes, skin and teeth, but also a receding of the upper lip and cracking of the skin, which bleeds when exposed to light. It has been suggested that physicians of the day could only treat sufferers by secluding them during the day and by persuading them to drink blood to replace that lost by bleeding (Illis, 1964:

[1]Formerly, Director, School of Social Work, Leicester University, England.

Milgrom, 1984; Prins, 1984). In more modern times, there have been accounts of people seeking to protect themselves from vampiric attentions (Farson & Hall, 1978).

There are also several quite well documented accounts of highly deviant individuals who were alleged to have indulged in vampiristic and necrophilic activities (Krafft-Ebing, 1978 and Summers, 1960). In 1827, Leger, aged 29 is alleged to have violated the corpse of a twelve and a half year old girl, mutilated her genitalia and drunk her blood. In the mid eighteen-forties, Sergeant Bertrand dug up corpses, sexually abused and mutilated them and then masturbated. He described himself as being in a state of great sexual excitement during these activities. Another Frenchman, Henri Blot, was tried in 1886 for necrophilia and vandalism. He had desecrated the grave of an eighteen year old girl and sexually abused her. Perhaps one of the most striking examples of this type of grossly abnormal behaviour is that shown by the notorious Peter Kurten in post World War I Germany. Kurten not only is alleged to have stabbed sheep whilst abusing them sexually but he also sexually mutilated and killed numerous men, women and children whilst allegedly indulging in necrophilic and vampiristic activities. Fritz Haarman, known as the 'Hanover vampire' (Summers, 1960), killed some twenty-four adolescent males. During the killings he indulged in vampiristic and necrophilic activity; Haarman was executed in 1925. In America, Albert Fish abducted a ten-year-old girl after killing her, cooked her flesh, consumed it, deriving sexual excitement from the activity. Finally, in this country, Haigh, the 'acid-bath' murderer has been considered by some authorities (Hemphill & Zabow, 1983) to have engaged in vampiristic activities. However, Hemphill & Zabow were possibly wrong in accepting Haigh's self-confessed vampiristic behaviour at face value (See also Neustatter, 1957: *Chapter XI*).

To gain some impression of the extent to which psychiatrists and certain other clinicians had come across such phenomena in their day-to-day work, information was obtained from some *fifty* respondents, mainly either forensic psychiatrists or psychiatrists with a particular interest in serious deviancy. They included three professors of forensic psychiatry, the medical directors of three special hospitals, and a senior officer of the Prison Medical Department. The sample is therefore very small, highly selective, and confined mainly (but not exclusively) to the United Kingdom; further details are given by Prins (1984). The survey revealed that blood ingestion in its various forms was a very uncommon phenomenon, which would perhaps account for the paucity of reported cases in the clinical literature. Thirty-three psychiatrist respondents suggested that any vampiristic activities they had come across were associated with other psychiatric disorders, and that vampirism was unlikely to constitute a single clinical entity. The psychiatric conditions that seemed to them to have the closest associations were, in order of frequency, schizophreniform disorders, hysteria, severe psychopathic disorder, and mental retardation. Hemphill & Zabow (1983) appear to limit their definition of clinical vampirism to blood ingestion, whereas other authorities (e.g. Bourguignon, 1983) include necrophilic activities which need not necessarily involve sexual intercourse. Bourguignon is at pains to point out that vampirism is a clinical phenomenon in which myth, fantasy, and reality converge. It should be noted here that the term 'vampirism' has also been used to include necrophagia and necrophilia as well as certain sadistic activities in relation to serious sexual assault, especially in those cases where frenzied sexual activity had taken place (Brittain, 1970). The word has also been used to include self/auto-vampirism.

CLASSIFICATION

From the information collected from respondents and from a synthesis of the sparse clinical literature, it is possible to suggest a four-fold classification:

1. Complete vampirism—involving ingestion of blood, necrophilic activity, and necro-sadism. This would also include what Walker (1978) has described as haemolagnia or blood lust (See also Burton-Bradley, 1976).
2. Vampirism without ingestion of blood or consumption of dead flesh. Bourguignon (1983) describes this as necrophilia pure and simple, and suggests that it consists of sexual satisfaction largely derived from touching (interference) or sexual intercourse with a dead body.
3. Vampirism without death being involved—see also Vandenberg & Kelly (1964), Krafft-Ebing, (1978), and Bourguignon, (1983).
4. Auto-vampirism. This heading would include those cases in which the individual derived satisfaction from ingestion

of his or her own blood (McCully, 1964, Hemphill & Zabow, 1983). The phenomenon of auto-vampirism can be further sub-divided into: (a) Self-induced bleeding with ingestion of blood. (b) Voluntary bleeding with re-ingestion of blood. (c) Auto-haemofetishism—a condition described by Bartholomew (1973) in which pleasure, mostly sexual, is derived from the sight of blood drawn up in a syringe in the process of intravenous drug addictive practice.

Some of the present author's respondents detailed cases in which self-mutilation had been linked with minor blood ingestive activity, most frequently in association with attention-seeking behaviour. Kwawer (1980) reports a serious example of this kind of self-mutilation: this concerned a female patient who stored her own blood in order to look at it in times of stress, since she considered it had a calming effect upon her. One of the author's respondents described a somewhat similar case in which a male patient stored his blood to achieve similar results.

AETIOLOGY

The literature on clinical vampirism seems to be very sparse, and this might well be because it is highly unlikely, even within a well-established therapeutic relationship, that a patient or offender will readily divulge information concerning vampiristic or similar activities. The phenomenon seems to exist alongside, or to be part of other clinical conditions. It is seen not infrequently in association with serious sexual offending, where biting and possibly the ingestion of blood may not be uncommon phenomena. It is interesting to speculate to what degree this behaviour is but a serious pathological extension of the normal and fairly common 'love-bite'. Some respondents suggested that vampiristic activities might well have their origins in, or be associated with schizophrenic processes, and several quoted instances in which paranoid patients had shown delusions of exsanguination. This would appear to be the equivalent of the "Psychic vampirism" described by Walker (1978). Incidents were also reported of auto-vampiristic activity; some of these were cases of mentally retarded patients who had also engaged in biting activity accompanied by minor blood ingestion. There are one or two cases reported in the clinical literature in which an hysterical state appears to have been associated with necrophilic activity, and Christie—the multiple killer—is sometimes regarded as an example of this association. It seems reasonable to speculate that such individuals can engage in their gruesome activities by a process akin to that of hysterical dissociation.

Whatever the cause or the form of its manifestation, vampiristic activity appears to occur in individuals functioning at a very primitive mental and emotional level. This may well explain the number of respondents who suggested the possible close connection between alleged clinical vampirism and *schizophrenic disorders.* Those who espouse a psychoanalytical view of aetiology would probably link such phenomena with the fantasies of biting and destruction seen in very small infants. Fenichel suggests that such persons, if fixated at a very early stage of development, may well become those leech-like individuals "who affix themselves . . . (to others) . . . by suction." (Fenichel, 1982, 489). Similar theoretical formulations have been propounded by Kayton (1972). Kwawer (1980), Benezech *et al* (1980, 1981) and Bourguignon (1983). A psychoanalytical conceptual framework would lead one to suggest that the schizophrenic, regressed schizoid, or 'borderline' individual has a compelling need to be provided for and to be nourished. The fear of exsanguination which has already been referred to may well be an extension of these needs in their severest presentation. This psychoanalytical view, incomplete and untestable though it may be in many respects, finds some degree of support in the clinical descriptions of some of the cases already mentioned. Vandenbergh & Kelly (1964) go so far as to suggest that the ingestion of blood may serve to satisfy very basic oral/sadistic needs.

CONCLUSION

On the basis of the available evidence, it would appear that vampirism as a single clinical condition is a most rare phenomenon. However, there are grounds for suggesting that it may be a more common phenomenon that has been supposed hitherto (Hemphill & Zabow, 1983). Further work could usefully be directed at making clearer the possible links between legendary and clinical phenomena: a Jungian conceptual framework might prove helpful in this respect. As McCully (1964) has suggested, "what lives in the forest beyond is shrouded in mist and as yet we have clumsy means to explore it". It is hoped that the foregoing modest contribution to the psychiatric literature will arouse or re-kindle interest in phenomena that transcend the fascinating boundaries between illness and evil and between myth and reality.

Criticism and comments from readers of the Journal would be welcomed by the author.

REFERENCES

Bartholomew, A. (1973) Two features occasionally associated with intravenous drug users: A note. *Australian and New Zealand Journal of Psychiatry,* 7. 1–2.

Benezech, M., Bourgeois, M., Villager, J. & Eichegaray, B. (1980) Cannibalizme et vampirisme chez un schizophrène multimeutrier. *Bordeaux Medical Journal*, 13, 1261–1265.

————Boukhabza, D. & Yesavage, J. (1981) Cannibalism and vampirism in paranoid schizophrenia. *Journal of Clinical Psychiatry,* 42, 290.

Bourguignon, A. (1983) Vampirism and autovampirism. In *Sexual Dynamics of Anti-Social Behaviour,* (eds. L. B. Schlesinger & E. Revitch). Chicago: Illinois: Charles C. Thomas.

Brittain, R. P. (1970) The sadistic murderer. *Medicine, Science and the Law,* 10, 198–207.

Burton-Bradley, B. G. (1976) *Cannibalism for cargo. The Journal of Nervous and Mental Disease*, 163, 428–431.

Farson, D. & Hall, J. (1978) *Mysterious Monsters.* (Enlarged edition). London: Aldus Books.

Fenichel, O. (1982) *The Psychoanalytic Theory of Neurosis.* London: Routledge & Kegan Paul.

Hemphill, R. E. & Zabow, T. (1983) Clinical vampirism: A presentation of three cases and a re-evaluation of Haigh the 'Acid-Bath Murderer'. *South African Medical Journal*, 63, 278–281.

Illis, L. (1964) On porphyria and the aetiology of werwolves. *Proceedings of the Royal Society of Medicine*. 57, 23–26.

Kayton, L. (1972) The relation of the vampire legend to schizophrenia. *Journal of Youth and Adolescence*. 1, 303–314.

Krafft-Ebing, R. von (1978) *Psychopathia Sexualis.* New York: Scarborough Books.

Kwawer, J. S. (1980) Some interpersonal aspects of self mutilation in a borderline patient. *Journal of the American Academy of Psychoanalysis*, 8, 203–216.

McCully, R. S. (1964) Vampirism: Historical perspective and underlying process in relation to a case of auto-vampirism. *Journal of Nervous and Mental Diseases*, 139, 440–452.

Milgrom, L. (1984) Vampires, plants and crazy kings. *New Scientists*. 26 April, 9–13.

Neustatter, W. L. (1957) *The Mind of the Murderer.* London: Christopher Johnson.

Prins, H. (1984) Vampirism—legendary or clinical phenomenon? *Medicine, Science and the Law,* 24, 283–293.

Summers, M. (1960) *The Vampire His Kith and Kin.* New York: University Books.

———(1980) *The Vampire in Europe.* Wellingborough: Aquarian Press.

Vandenbergh, R. L. & Kelly, J. R. (1964) Vampirism: A review with new observations. *Archives of General Psychiatry.* 11, 543–547.

Walker, R. (1978) *Encyclopaedia of Metaphysical Medicine.* London: Routledge & Kegan Paul.

PART II

LYCANTHROPY

"The heart of man is the place the Devil dwells in: I feel sometimes a hell within myself."

Sir Thomas Browne,
Religio Medici, 1643

Introduction

"*Lycanthropia*: a Madness proceeding from a Mad wolf, wherein Men imitate the howling of Wolves."

Stephen Blancard,
A Physical Dictionary. . . . 1684

"It's when I was bitten by a rabid dog. . . . When I'm emotionally upset, I feel as if I'm turning into something else. . . . I get the feeling I'm becoming a wolf. I look at myself in the mirror and I witness my transformation. It's no longer my face; it changes completely. I stare, my pupils dilate, and I feel as if hairs are growing all over my body, as if my teeth are getting longer. . . . I feel as if my skin is no longer 'mine."

"Mr. A.," a 28-year-old
French lycanthrope, 1989

LYCANTHROPY: AN ANCIENT AFFLICTION

The above definition of lycanthropy from Stephen Blancard (1650–1702) comes from the very first medical dictionary ever published in the English language, a translation of Blancard's (sometimes spelled Blankaart's) Latin original of 1679. Medical descriptions of a mental disorder known as lycanthropy or lycanthropia date back at least to the writings of Marcellus of Side (A.D. ?–161), and the cluster of signs and symptoms that he describes was passed down through the centuries in its essential form by one medical commentator after another for the next 1600 years. However, a 1990s medical dictionary entry for lycanthropy would not read much differently, as is illustrated by the quote from the case history of the lycanthropic murder reported by the

French authority on lycanthropy, psychiatrist Michel Benezech, and his colleagues (Benezech et al., 1989).

The essential feature of this disorder is the notion of a human taking the form of a wolf and then literally behaving like one (transforming into other animals such as dogs and cats is also not uncommon). Although originally viewed as only a mental disorder, during the period of the Great Witch Hunt in Europe (roughly 1500–1650), such individuals were regarded as instruments of Satan, and many were executed as lycanthropes (or *loups garoux* in France), for changing their forms with the Devil's help—that is, literally transforming themselves into animals—and then committing heretical or violent crimes. Many persons actually believed that lycanthropes or "werewolves" truly enacted this miraculous physical transformation. Others believed it was merely a delusion, but during Europe's dark struggle with witchcraft, many believed that even if lycanthropy was delusional in nature the delusion had been put in the afflicted person's mind by Satan and he or she should be tried and put to death anyway. The most important of the many Inquisitorial trials for lycanthropy during this period, particularly in France, are summarized according to their various subject entries in an invaluable book by Robbins (1959). The use of magical "ointments" that allowed witches to fly to the Sabbat was also implicated in many accounts of men transforming into wolves or other animals, leading to the suspicion by post-Psychedelic Era scholars such as anthropologist Michael Harner (1973) that the ingestion or absorption of hallucinogenic substances was at the root of these experiences. As the witch trials began to subside in the 17th century, the medical model definition of lycanthropy returned, resembling in many respects the descriptions of the ancients.

LYCANTHROPE AND WEREWOLF

In English, the words lycanthrope and werewolf are often used interchangeably. The word "werewolf" makes its first appearance in English in the ecclesiastical ordinances of King Canute sometime between A.D. 1017 and 1035. However, its use in the Old Teutonic languages dates back to a much earlier period. The word *were*, or *wer*, is the Old English word for man, and it is a derivative of the Latin word for man, *vir*. Therefore, a werewolf is literally a man-wolf, or, in the archaic spelling of England's King James I in his treatise *Daemonologie* (Edinburgh,

1597), a "Man-Woolfe." Lycanthrope comes from two Greek words that mean wolf-man. The first time the term *lycanthropy* made its appearance in an English language publication was in Reginald Scot's book, *The Discoverie of Witchcraft* (London, 1584), and it was used in its current sense, to refer to a mental disorder.

As is true of vampirism, lycanthropy is likewise both a clinical and a legendary phenomenon. However, over the centuries a certain convention has developed in the English language about the use of the words lycanthropy and werewolfism, or lycanthropes and werewolves. The word lycanthropy is generally used in discussions of the clinical nature of this phenomenon, whereas in the areas of folklore or myths and legends involving the actual physical shape-shifting of an individual, it is more likely that werewolves will be discussed. Or, because so many persons were called werewolves who committed atrocities during the Middle Ages and the Renaissance (the equivalent of our modern-day serial killers, mass murderers, or persons who commit the sort of crimes described by Krafft-Ebing as "lust-murders"), this term is still commonly used to refer to these sadistic criminals as well. An insightful psychological interpretation of the legendary werewolf is provided by author Anne Rice in a review that appeared in *The New York Times Book Review*:

> I would like to suggest that the werewolf in many instances embodies a potent blending of masochistic and sadistic elements. On the one hand, man is degraded as he is forced to submit to the bestial metamorphosis; on the other hand, he emerges as a powerful sadistic predator who can, without regret, destroy other men. The werewolf as both victim and victimizer, wrapped in magic, may arouse emotions in us that are hard to define. (Rice, 1987)

The vast literature on the folklore of the werewolf and its many representations in literature and in motion pictures need not be discussed here. The best—and again, the most quirky—compilation of cross-cultural scholarly materials on the legend of the werewolf is the book by Montague Summers (1933). Summers believes in the reality of werewolves and insists that they are the agents of Satan. His chilling chapter, "The Werewolf: His Science and Practice" compiles evidence for the satanic nature of this creature. However, he does make the distinction that lycanthropes are truly mentally ill and delusional and that werewolves actually do shape-shift into other animals. Unfortunately, Summers then regresses to 16th century logic by arguing that because lycanthropy is a mental disorder, and all mental disorders are in fact caused by diabolical possession, that persons with lycanthropy are diabolically possessed and therefore the unwitting agents of the Devil(!). If the seriousness with which he makes these statements is genuine, then Summers would have made a superb exterminator of hundreds of fellow humans if he had just been born a few centuries earlier.

An exemplary collection of excerpts and full primary documents relating to lycanthropy and werewolfism has been gathered and published by Charlotte Otten (1987). Otten (whose book Anne Rice was reviewing above), a professor of English, brings together for the first time primary resources on lycanthropy and werewolfism from medicine, jurisprudence, history, philosophy, theology, mythology, and folklore. Although dwarfed by Summers' erudition, Otten's book is the first place to turn for a credible treatment of the subject. Devlin (1987, pp. 72–80) examines the superstitious beliefs of 18th and 19th century French peasants concerning "werewolves and monsters" in another scholarly volume. In a more popular treatment, Dracula scholar Raymond T. McNally (1983) links the folklore of the werewolf to the vampire legend and necrophilia in attempting to understand the gruesome life of mass murderess Elisabeth Bathory, the 16th century "Blood Countess" of Hungary. Less readily available sources about werewolves are the rare volumes by Herz (1862) and Black (1920).

The idea that humans transform themselves into wolves may date back at least 2700 years. The ancient Greek roots of werewolves are traced by the German classical scholar Walter Burkert in his classic book, *Homo Necans: The Anthropology of Ancient Greek Sacrificial Ritual and Myth* (1972/1983, pp. 84-93). Burkert argues the case for rituals involving animal and human sacrifice during secret nocturnal festivals that were held at the ash-altar of the sanctuary of Zeus Lykaios in Arcadia, perhaps as far back as 700 B.C. Men would be transformed into wolves after eating the mixture of human and animal entrails from a large tripod kettle. Although Burkert (p. 90) admits that modern archeologists still have not found human bones during excavations on the site at Mount Lykion, he still believes the ancient Greeks maintained a cult of werewolves based on cannibalistic rituals, as is found in the more recent ethnographic examples of secret societies of "leopard men" or "tiger men" in Africa and Asia. "There is no doubt that werewolves existed, just like leopard men and tiger men, as a clandestine *Männerbund,* a secret society, wavering between demonic possession and horseplay, as is common in such a *Männerbund.*" (Burkert, 1972/1983, p. 88).

In later periods, certain regions of Europe—particularly the Balto-Slavic areas—seem to have been particularly associated with the belief in werewolves. In the highly regarded work on Indo-European language and culture, Mallory (1989, p.83) repeats the story by a skeptical Herodotus that a 6th century B.C. Baltic tribe known as the Neuri transformed themselves into werewolves one or two days a year. As Maia Madar (1990), a researcher at the Historical Institute of the Estonian Academy of Sciences, has documented, the ancient Baltic region of Livonia or Livland (now modern Estonia) was a hotbed of werewolf activity. In the 1600s, as part of the larger phenomenon of witch trials, at least 31 men and women were brought to trial for causing damage to property, animals, or other people while transformed into werewolves. Additional Baltic reports of *Wahrwolf* activity can be found in the obscure study by von Bruiningk (1924–1928).

Humans did not just transform themselves into wolves (lycanthropy), they also transformed themselves into dogs (cyanthropy). The figure of the "dog-man" has appeared in many myths in many cultures, and these myths of the dog-man have been extensively documented in an exemplary study by White (1991).

LYCANTHROPY, MELANCHOLIA, ZOANTHROPY

It is remarkable that in the 1800-year history of the mental disorder we continue to call lycanthropy, we can still read the clinical descriptions of the ancients and recognize certain rare 20th century individuals (such as those in the case histories reprinted in this section). Because the 2nd century fragments of Marcellus of Side's writings on lycanthropy have never been translated from the original Greek into English, many scholars commonly cite the description provided by Paul of Aegina (625–690), which was based on Marcellus' work. Besides being the most detailed description available in English, the work of Paul of Aegina is important because it was the first to link lycanthropy with melancholy, an association that would last until the 19th century.

In the 1844 translation by Francis Adams, Paul describes this mental disorder in the following way:

> On Lycaon, or Lycanthropia. Those laboring under lycanthropia go out during the night imitating wolves in all things and lingering about sepulchers until morning. You may recognize such persons by these marks: they are pale, their vision feeble, their eyes dry, tongue very dry, and the flow of the saliva stopped; but they are thirsty, and their legs have incurable ulcerations from frequent falls. Such are the marks of the disease. You must know that lycanthropia is a species of melancholy which you may cure at the time of the attack, by opening a vein and abstracting blood to fainting, and giving the patient a diet of wholesome food. Let him use baths of sweet water, and then milk-whey for three days, and purging with the hiera from colocynth twice or thrice. After the purgings use the theriac of vipers, and administer those things mentioned for the cure of melancholy. . . . When the disease is already formed, use soporific embrocations, and rub the nostrils with opium when going to rest. (Adams, 1844, III, pp. 389–390)

In his discussion of lycanthropy, Harner (1973, p. 141) points out that the symptoms described in this passage "closely resemble those reported for the clinical effects of atropine," an hallucinogenic substance that Harner argues was used in European witchcraft to deliberately induce visionary altered states of consciousness. The use of hallucinogens by some 20th century lycanthropes prior to the onset of their symptoms are described in the two case reports below by psychiatrists F. G. Surawicz and R. Banta, whose 1975 article in the *Canadian Psychiatric Association Journal* ignited modern interest in this archaic disorder.

An exemplary summary of the nosological history of lycanthropy within medicine and psychiatry is provided in the important volume by psychiatrist Stanley W. Jackson, *Melancholia and Depression: From Hippocratic Times to Modern Times* (1986). In his chapter on "Lycanthropy" (pp. 345–351), Jackson points out that during the witch hunts of the Renaissance, the disorder took on more characteristics of mania than of melancholia in the minds of many theological and legal authorities, relating it to demoniacal possession and thus the influence of the Devil. But by the middle of the 17th century, Jackson claims, lycanthropy was once again viewed as a species of melancholia—just as it originally had been. During the latter part of the 17th century and the eighteenth century, Jackson reports that lycanthropy "gradually became less prominent in medical writings." The sporadic discussions of lycanthropy by medical authorities would sometimes result in new names for the disorder: "*rabies Hydrophobica*" by Stephen Blankaart in 1679; "*melancholia zoantropia*" by Francois Boissier de Sauvages in 1770; "*zoantropic melancholia*" by Thomas Cullen in 1793, who also included a category for the delusion of being transformed into a horse, "*hippantropic melancholia*"; a form of "sensitive insanity" by Thomas Arnold in 1806; "*melancholia metamorphosis*" by Johann Christian Heinroth at about the same time; and "*zoanthropy*" by J.E.D. Esquirol in 1838. Jackson (1986) closes his summary with the conclusion that, "As these brief references suggest, lycanthropy had essentially disappeared as a syndrome, and there was no tendency for it to return in the nosologies of the late nineteenth and twentieth centuries" (p. 350).

However, this state of affairs may change. Since 1975, a total of 18 new cases of lycanthropy have been reported in English and French language psychiatric journals in eight different publications (Surawicz and Banta, 1975; Rosenstock, 1977; Jackson, 1978; Coll et al., 1985; Keck et al., 1988; Benezech et al., 1988, 1989, Kulick et al., 1990). Of these 18 cases, six were transformed into wolves, four were dogs (a common variant known as cyanthropy), two were cats, and the rest included a tiger, a gerbil, a rabbit, and two unspecified animals. Due to the fine research of French psychiatrists H. Verdoux, J. de Witt, M. Benezech, and M. Bourgeois (1989), three 19th century case histories from France have been discovered (Bariod, 1850; Morel, 1853; Stahl, 1873), all of whom were transformed into wolves.

It is interesting that in the more than 100 years between 1873 and 1975, the only published report of a case of lycanthropy that has surfaced to date is a case mentioned briefly in an essay by C.G. Jung published in 1928. Jung includes the case of lycanthropy in his essay as an example of how sensitive children are to the unconscious dynamics of their parents:

> I remember a very revealing case of three girls who had a *most* devoted mother. When they were approaching puberty

> they confessed shamefacedly to each other that for years they had suffered from horrible dreams about her. They dreamt of her as a witch or a dangerous animal, and they could not understand it at all, since their mother was so lovely and so utterly devoted to them. Years later the mother became insane, and in her insanity would exhibit a sort of lycanthropy in which she crawled about on all fours and imitated the grunting of pigs, the barking of dogs, and the growling of bears. (Jung, 1928/1954, p. 55)

Of all the various standard psychiatric diagnoses given to these individuals, bipolar disorder is the most common (8 of the 12 in the series by Keck and his colleagues, reprinted in this volume), followed by schizophrenia (3); pseudoneurotic schizophrenia (1); delusional depression (1); major depression (1); chronic brain syndrome (1); schizoid personality traits (1); borderline personality disorder (1); and depersonalization disorder (1).

Perhaps, following the lead of the French psychiatric literature, this clinical phenomenon should be more correctly referred to as zoanthropy, the delusion that one has been transformed into an animal, with lycanthropy being reserved for the traditional wolf distinction, cyanthropy for dogs, and so on. This would prove to be of great value in including case histories from non-Western sources, such as cases of Kitsune-Tsuki syndrome from Japan in which people believe they are possessed by malevolent foxes and act like them (Furukawa & Bourgeois, 1984).

IS ZOANTHROPY A DISSOCIATIVE DISORDER?

There are several interesting parallels between the history of lycanthropy (zoanthropy) as a mental disorder and its presenting symptoms and the history and symptoms of a dissociative disorder that is also currently much in vogue, multiple personality disorder.

First, both disorders suddenly reappeared in the mid-1970s after decades of presumed extinction. Between 1910 and 1975 very few cases of multiple personality disorder were reported in the psychiatric literature due, it is suggested by some, to the acceptance of Eugen Bleuler's broader diagnostic criteria for dementia praecox (schizophrenia), which means that such cases may have been misdiagnosed therefore as schizophrenia. The same may be true of cases of zoanthropy, although they may have been subsumed under other diagnoses (e.g., monomania, hysteria, paranoia, etc.) practically since the first beginnings of psychiatry as a profession in the early 1800s. The reason that both multiple personality disorder and zoanthropy seemed to resurface in the psychiatric literature at about the same time is that clinicians were improving their understanding of dissociative phenomena of all types and were learning to distinguish these signs and symptoms from those of other diagnostic categories.

Second, zoanthropes report a significant disturbance or alteration in the normally integrative functions of identity and consciousness, and possibly even memory, although this hypothesis remains to be investigated. These disturbances are the hallmark of the dissociative disorders.

Third, the transformation of human into animal may be analogous to the "switching" process observed in persons with multiple personality disorder in which the personality in executive control of the body is replaced by another. This may mean that some cases of zoanthropy may actually be manifestations of multiple personality disorder, or they may fit the category of "dissociative disorder not otherwise specified" if the animal ego-state never assumes complete control.

Fourth, persons with multiple personality disorder can have nonhuman alternate personalities, and the zoanthropic behaviors may simply be alternate personalities. One such case involving animal alters is reported by Smith (1989), and additional cases have been provided by Hendrickson, McCarty, and Goodwin (1990), although their psychopathological interpretation of "the animal familiars of witches and shamans" (p. 220) is a gross misconception based on an ignorance of the historical and ethnographic literatures relating to those subjects. Nonhuman alters are acknowledged as present in some MPD patients in the textbooks of two major authorities in the field, Putnam (1989) and Ross (1989).

Fifth, MPD is often misdiagnosed, and the most common wrong diagnoses are given to those cases listed above with zoanthropy. Indeed, the very fact that there is so much disagreement over diagnostic categories across cases may indicate that something else, such as a dissociative disorder, may be present in cases of zoanthropy. The extensive case history of the 26-year-old "cat man" with the recalcitrant zoanthropy reported by Kulick et al. (1990) has many of the indications of possible MPD: childhood abuse (confinement—tied to a tree for hours until school age); a secret cat identity; multiple episodes of severe depression; one suicide attempt; lifelong daily or weekly "absence" spells, which diminished in frequency after age 21; visual distortions; episodes of déjà vu that occurred weekly, and so on. All of these are strong indications that a dissociative disorder may be present.

THE BEAST WITHIN US ALL

Like vampirism, lycanthropy is a clinical phenomenon in which myth, fantasy, and reality converge. What needs to be addressed is the psychological significance of the peculiar form that the symptoms of this disorder manifests—the transformation of humans into animals.

Throughout history, the legend of the lycanthrope or werewolf has symbolized the dual nature of humankind—the interplay of our spiritual and carnal natures, the struggle between the sacred and profane within the human soul. The primal, bestial side of the human animal is in evidence in the darker urges within us all. Those who refuse to obey the rules of the greater society may choose to act out the impulses of animals: to rape, to murder, to mutilate, to cannibalize.

Generally, in our "civilized" society, anything that reminds us of our animal natures tends to be suppressed. Unlike other societies, particularly nonliterate ones in which the adoption of animal identities may be a part of the normal process of ego development, in our culture we are taught to dissociate ourselves from our baser instincts, to remind ourselves that we are not animals but creatures of a higher order. Yet the urges are present: sex, aggression, hunger, thirst, and so on. Their presence reminds us of a different truth. It is no wonder, then, that so many persons are conflicted about these very issues and experience extreme difficulties with their sexuality, with expressing anger (too much or too little), with aberrant eating patterns (anorexia, bulimia, obesity), with alcoholism and other drug addictions. When we dissociate too severely from the animal within us all, the biological imperative of human existence, by not allowing its expression in fantasy or behavior and accepting our dual natures, then we pay dearly for it in terms of our emotional and physical health.

According to C.G. Jung (1947/1969), the "dissociability of the psyche" is a fundamental psychological process that extends along the continuum from "normal" mental functioning to "abnormal" mental states. From Jung's perspective, as so many of the features of our animal nature are often unacceptable to us, it is natural that they are suppressed from awareness through a dissociative process. These split-off streams of consciousness form complexes, nodal points or clusters of affect whose dynamics are observed in the phenomenon we term personality. Jung felt that the ego (also sometimes referred to by Jung as the ego-complex or ego-consciousness) was the most important of the complexes since it derived primarily from the somatic memory traces from the earliest years of life, was associated with the birth name, and was primarily the center of consciousness in "normals."

However, Jung stresses repeatedly in his phenomenological analysis of consciousness that the ego is only one of many autonomous complexes, each with an allotment of consciousness all its own, which interact and often conflict with the ego for executive control of conscious processes and the body. In pathological conditions, such as multiple personality disorder, schizophrenia and, presumably, zoanthropy, their strength is greater and their dissociation from the ego more extreme, disabling the personality with "a multiplication of its centers of gravity" (Jung, 1946/1966 p. 173). Therefore, Jung often calls complexes "splinter psyches" (Jung, 1934/1969, p. 97).

Jung observed that the psyche splits in typical patterns, and he referred to the unconscious underlying organizational factors of the psyche as archetypes. A point I made in an earlier paper (Noll, 1989) with reference to the relevance of Jung's complex theory to the study of multiple personality disorder is that "Jung's early phenomenological method may have uncovered *typical patterns of dissociation* and the subsequent *personification of autonomous psychic factors* that are now once again being studied with a quantitative scientific methodology" (p. 365). One such autonomous factor that has a special relationship to "the beast within us all" is the archetype Jung calls the *shadow.*

Jung (1951/1968, p. 266) defines the shadow as "that hidden, repressed, for the most part inferior and guilt-laden personality whose ultimate ramifications reach back into the realm of our animal ancestors and so comprise the whole historical aspect of the unconscious." Elsewhere Jung (1955/1970, p. 253) says, "The shadow is the primitive who is still alive and active in civilized man, and our civilized reason means nothing to him." The various dissociations that produce complexes can sometimes be related to the archetype of the shadow. For example, in multiple personality disorder, the shadow may be represented by persecutor personalities, homicidal or suicidal alters, personalities claiming to be demons or the devil, or personalities with impulse control problems who wildly act out episodes of sexual promiscuity, substance abuse, and sociopathy.

If the attempts to prevent shadow complexes from assimilating into the ego-complex result in a strong dissociation, with the goal of trying to separate and compartmentalize this material and keep it from ever entering consciousness by the construction of an amnesic barrier, then the autonomy of the split-off ego states or alternate personalities becomes stronger, and the shadow may even take on bestial form in the dreams and fantasies of an individual. Perhaps the best literary example of this can be found in Robert Louis Stevenson's book *Dr. Jekyll and Mr. Hyde*, published in 1886. Dr. Henry Jekyll, a moral and well-respected physician, decides that the world would be a much better place if humans could separate their innate goodness from their innate evilness, for as Dr. Jekyll writes in the "full statement of the case" he left behind,

> It was the curse of mankind that these incongruous faggots were thus bound together—that in the agonised womb of consciousness, these polar twins should be continually struggling. How, then, were they dissociated? (Stevenson, 1886/1981, p. 80)

Jekyll invents a drug that will dissociate him into his good and evil parts. He takes the drug with the result that not only an emotional but a psychological and a physical transformation takes place. His dissociated dark half becomes fully autonomous and claims an identity for itself in the form of Edward Hyde. Furthermore, when the drug transforms Jekyll into his dark alter ego, he becomes, in the words of the lawyer Utterson who once saw him, "hardly human," "pale and dwarfish," "troglodytic," and he gives off "an impression of deformity without any nameable malformation." Jekyll is able to control the strength of the dissociation at first, but soon Hyde becomes more autonomous and Jekyll is terrified when he finds himself transforming into this "brute" without warning. Jekyll's attempts to separate himself from his shadow only make Hyde more autonomous and Jekyll more vulnerable to his dark influences.

Hyde (as perhaps even the name suggests) is more animal than human. He is violent toward children, it is hinted that he rapes, and he murders brutally and joyfully. Jekyll's description of his unsolicited transformation into this brute is similar to the reported experiences of the 20th century lycanthropes included in this volume, and it is indeed not surprising that motion picture images of Edward Hyde depict him as resembling a werewolf. As Jekyll writes to his lawyer in a final posthumous statement:

> Now the hand of Henry Jekyll (as you have often remarked) was professional in shape and size: it was large, firm, white and comely. But the hand which I now saw . . . was lean, corded, knuckly, of a dusky pallor and thickly shaded with a swart growth of hair. It was the hand of Edward Hyde. (Stevenson, 1886/1981, p. 88)

The belief that an alternate animal identity exists in all humans (and that it is connected in some way with notions of "evil") finds some support in the ethnographic literature as well. Some examples are provided in the section on "The Human and the Animal," an extensive ethnographic literature review that can be found in the often-cited volume *African Leopard Men* by Lindskog (1954). A more detailed example is provided, in Ruel's (1970) study of the Banyang of the Cameroon in Africa, in which he described the societal belief that "people can change into or can send out 'animals' and that it is these animals that carry out the evil (witchcraft) intentions of their owners" (Ruel, 1970, p. 334). It is not only witches who have this ability, however, for as Ruel (1970) explains:

> A 'were-person' or witch (*me debu*) can be referred to in general terms as an evil or deceitful person, but it is also understood that all human beings have in some form 'were-animals' (*babu*), and there is indeed a great range of named were-animals that people are said to possess. Moreover, this range of were-animals extends from those that are the most evil, the most perverted in their abilities, to those that are entirely unreprehensible and appear sometimes as little more than metaphorical descriptions of a person's individual talents. Again, one person may possess a number of were-animals,

> drawn from different points on the total range, which determine as it were his 'complexion' as a were-owner. (p. 334)

Like the case reports of zoanthropy and the fictional example of Henry Jekyll and Edward Hyde, Ruel says that among the Banyang, "in most cases the were-animal or were-type is in some sense a 'double' or alternative identity of the person who owns it." However, unlike our cultural examples, "the area in which it moves is again a 'double' world, another existence parallel to the actual world (*kekepe*) in which people live" (Ruel, 1970, 335). However, following Jung's phenomenology, this idea is congruent with his idea of the shadow as an archetype of the collective unconscious, a separate world outside the range of direct observation of consciousness.

If zoanthropy is a dissociative disorder (from our culture's point of view), then the split-off alter egos may be related to the realm of human experience Jung identifies as that of the shadow. The phenomenology of the shadow is represented in the following characteristics of the lycanthropes' case histories presented in this volume, through which the bestial and evil or satanic nature of their alter egos is manifested. These reported traits (which also resemble the ancient accounts) are:

1. The belief that they are wolves, dogs, or other animals and that they have been physically transformed into these animals, even to the point of experiencing the growth of fur, claws, or fangs.
2. Animal-like behavior, including growling, howling, clawing, pawing, crawling on all fours, and animal-like sexual behaviors.
3. The desire to assault or kill others, or actually doing so.
4. Hypersexuality, including the desire to have sex with animals (bestiality).
5. The use of hallucinogenic or other substances to achieve the metamorphosis of human into wolf.
6. A desire for isolation from human society (stalking the woods, haunting cemeteries).
7. The belief that the devil or some evil or satanic force is behind the transformation of human into animal form.

Not every case exhibits all of these traits, but most exhibit one or more of them. Lycanthropy is indeed alive and well in the 20th century—as is the shadow.

REFERENCES

Adams, F. (1844). *The Seven Books of Paulus Aegineta*. 3 vols. London: The Sydenham Society.

Bariod, A. (1850). Observation d'un cas de lycanthropie. *Annales Médico-Psychologique*, 151–154.

Benezech, M. (1988) Médico-diableries nocturnes. *Practicien du Sud-Ouest*, 2, 16–17, 5–6.

Benezech, M., De Witte, J., Etchepare, J. J., & Bourgeois, M. (1988). A propos d'une onservation de lycanthropie avec violences mortelles. *Annales Médico-Psychologique*, 464–470.

Benezech, M., De Witte, J., Etcheparre, J. J., & Bourgeois, M. (1989). A lycanthropic murderer. *American Journal of Psychiatry. 146*, 942.

Black, G. (1920). *A List of Works Relating to Lycanthropy*. New York: Public Library.

Boulhaut, J.P. (1988). Lycanthropie et pathologie mentale. *Thesis:* University of Bordeaux II, No. 179, 65 pp.

Burkert, W. (1972/1983). *Homo Necans: The Anthropology of Ancient Greek Sacrificial Ritual and Myth*. P. Bing (translator). Berkley: University of California Press.

Coll, P.G., O'Sullivan, G., & Browne, P.J. (1985). Lycanthropy lives on. *British Journal of Psychiatry, 147*, 201–202.

Devlin, J. (1987). *The Superstitious Mind: French Peasants and the Supernatural in the Nineteenth Century*. New Haven: Yale University Press.

Furukawa, F., & Bourgeois, M. (1984). Délire de possession par le renard au Japon (ou délire de Kitsune-Tsuki). *Annales Médico-Psychologique. 142*, 5, 677–687.

Harner, M. (1973). The role of hallucinogenic plants in European witchcraft. In M. Harner (Ed.), *Hallucinogens and Shamanism*. New York: Oxford University Press.

Hendrickson, K.M., McCarty, T., & Goodwin, J. M. (1990). Animal alters: Case reports. *Dissociation, 3*, 218–221.

Herz, W. (1862). *Der Werewolf.* Stuttgart.

Jackson, P.M. (1978). Another case of lycanthropy. *American Journal of Psychiatry*, 134–135.

Jackson, S.W. (1986). *Melancholia and Depression: From Hippocratic Times to Modern Times*. New Haven: Yale University Press.

Jung, C.G. (1928/1954). Child development and education. In Jung, C.G., *The Development of Personality. The Collected Works of C.G. Jung, Vol. 17*. Princeton: Princeton University Press.

Jung, C.G. (1934/1969). A review of the complex theory. In Jung, C.G., *The Structure and Dynamics of the Psyche. The Collected Works of C.G. Jung, Vol. 8*. Princeton: Princeton University Press.

Jung, C.G. (1946/1966). The psychology of the transference. In Jung, C.G., *The Practice of Psychotherapy. The Collected Works of C.G. Jung, Vol. 16*. Princeton: Princeton University Press.

Jung, C.G. (1947/1954/1969). On the nature of the psyche. In Jung. C.G., *The Structure and Dynamics of the Psyche. The Collected Works of C.G. Jung, Vol. 8*. Princeton: Princeton University Press.

Jung, C.G. (1951/1968). *Aion: Researches into the Phenomenology of the Self. The Collected Works of C.G. Jung, Vol. 9, II*. Princeton: Princeton University Press.

Jung, C.G. (1955/1970). *Mysterium Conjunctionis. The Collected Works of C.G. Jung, Vol. 14*. Princeton: Princeton University Press.

Keck, P.E., Pope, H.G., Hudson, J.I., McElroy, S.L., & Kulick, A.R. (1988). Lycanthropy: Alive and well in the twentieth century. *Psychological Medicine, 18*, 113–120.

Kulick, A.R., Pope, H.G., & Keck, P.E. (1990). Lycanthropy and self-identification. *Journal of Nervous and Mental Disease, 178*, 134–137.

Lindskog, B. (1954). *African Leopard Men*. Uppsala: Studia Ethnographica Upsaliensia VII.

Madar, M. (1990). Estonia I: Werewolves and poisoners. In B. Ankarloo & G. Henningsen (Eds.), *Early Modern European Witchcraft*. Oxford: Clarendon Press.

Mallory, J.P. (1989). *In Search of the Indo-Europeans: Language, Archeology and Myth*. London: Thames & Hudson.

McNally, R.T. (1983). *Dracula Was a Woman: In Search of the Blood Countess of Transylvania*. New York: McGraw-Hill.

Morel, B.A. (1853). *Traité théorique et pratique des maladies mentales*. Paris: Masson. (T.1, pp. 263–265, T.2, pp. 58–59.)

Noll, R. (1989). Multiple personality, dissociation, and C.G. Jung's complex theory. *Journal of Analytical Psychology, 34*, 353–370.

Otten, C.F. (Ed.) (1987). *A Lycanthropy Reader: Werewolves in Western Culture*. Syracuse, NY: Syracuse University Press.

Putnam, F.W. (1989). *Diagnosis and Treatment of Multiple Personality Disorder*. New York: Guilford.

Rice, A. (April 5, 1987). Whither the werewolf. *The New York Times Book Review*, p. 33.

Robbins, R.H. (1959). *The Encyclopedia of Witchcraft and Demonology*. New York: Crown.

Rosenstock, H.A., & Vincent, K.R. (1977). A case of lycanthropy. *American Journal of Psychiatry, 134*, 1147–1149.

Ross, C.A. (1989). *Multiple Personality Disorder: Diagnosis, Clinical Features, and Treatment*. New York: John Wiley & Sons.

Ruel, Malcom. (1970) Were-animals and the introverted witch. In M. Douglas (Ed.), *Witchcraft Confessions and Accusations*. London: Tavistock.

Smith, S.G. (1989). Multiple personality disorder with human and non-human subpersonality components. *Dissociation, 2*, 52–57.

Stahl, A. (1873). Un cas de lycanthropie. *Annales Médico-Psychologique, 13*, 455.

Stevenson, R.L. (1886/1981). *Dr. Jekyll and Mr. Hyde*. New York: Bantam.

Summers, M. (1933). *The Werewolf*. London: Routledge.

Surawicz, F.A., & Banta, R. (1975). Lycanthropy revisited. *Canadian Psychiatric Association Journal, 20*, 537–542.

Verdoux, H., de Witt, J., Benezech, M., & Bourgeois, M. (1989). La lycanthropie: Une pathologie contemporaine? *Annales de Psychiatrie, 4*, 175–179.

von Bruiningk, H. (1924–1928). Der Werwolf in Livland und das letzte im Wendeschen Landgericht und Dörptschen Hofgericht i. J. 1692 deshalb stattgehabte Strafverfahren. *Mitteilungen aus der livländischen Geschichte, 22*.

White, D. (1991). *Myths of the Dog-Man*. Chicago: University of Chicago Press.

6

Lycanthropy Revisited

FRIDA G. SURAWICZ, *M.D.*[1]
RICHARD BANTA, *M.D.*[2]

Most contemporary textbooks, with the exception of the *American Handbook of Psychiatry* (1) do not mention the term lycanthropy—the delusion of being changed into a wolf. Recently, two patients with symptoms of this disorder were admitted and studied on an inpatient service. Their cases are reported here because of the unusual symptomatology of this allegedly extinct condition.

REVIEW OF LITERATURE

The literature on lycanthropy is extensive and includes publications from ancient as well as modern times. It is widespread across the world. The near extinction of wolves in Western Europe and most of America may well have diminished the occurrence of lycanthropy in the Western World but the condition continues to exist in a modified form in China, India, Indonesia, Assam, Malaysia, and in many African countries.[2,3] In these countries, the delusions include transformation into other ferocious animals, such as hyenas, tigers, crocodiles, and wolves.

[1]Associate Professor, Department of Psychiatry, University of Kentucky Medical College; Chief of Psychiatry, Veterans Administration Hospital, Lexington, Kentucky.
[2]Resident in Psychiatry, University of Kentucky Medical College.

Reprinted with permission from *Canadian Psychiatric Association Journal*, 1975, Vol. 20, 537–542.

The definition of lycanthropy through the ages is fairly universal, namely that once a man is changed into a wolf, he acquires its characteristics, roaming around at night, howling in cemeteries and attacking man or beast in search of raw flesh. However, there have always been two interpretations of this condition, often diametrically opposed.

The religious interpretation, based on mythology and superstition, sees the metamorphosis of man into wolf either as a divine punishment or as the outcome of a pact with the devil. This interpretation was first recorded in Greek mythology, when Lycaon, a tyrant in Arcadia, in order to test Zeus, secretly fed him the flesh of a slayed Molossian. Zeus became outraged, destroyed Lycaon's palace and transformed him into a howling wolf.[4,5] Medieval and Renaissance theologians thought that werewolfism could be caused by the evil eye or by satanic ointments. Jean Bodin, a sixteenth century French physician, states that ". . . the devil can really and materially metamorphose the body of a man into that of an animal and thereby cause the sickness".[6] In the twentieth century, Montague Summers believes firmly in werewolfism, and traces it back to an ancient cult connected with the Baal religion and probably imported by a Phoenician race in the former Arcadia in Greece, where wolves and the devil presumably were worshipped in high places and received human sacrifices.[7]

In contrast, scientists and physicians from antiquity on have seen lycanthropy as a form of disease, either a type of melancholia with delirium, or drug induced. These viewpoints were expressed by Marcellus Sidetes,[8] Galen[1] and Vergil.[9] After the Middle Ages and under the influence of the Inquisition, many scientists and physicians took a compromise position. Sennert felt that lycanthropy is a disease which can be brought upon one by means of spells and black magic, by a glance of the evil eye or by muttering some occult rune. He stated that the devil uses poisons which can heighten or aggravate natural diseases and that he can torment man by causing madness.[10] Peter Thyraeus explained the metamorphosis of man into wolf in three ways—it can be caused by hallucinations, or an animal form can be superimposed upon the human form, or a person can be cast into a slumber or trance by the devil, whereupon the astral body is clothed with an animal form.[11] In contrast to these ambiguous positions, Donato Antonio Altomari, a physician in sixteenth century Naples, wrote that lycanthropy is indeed a disease predominantly occurring in February, characterized by excessive thirst and complete loss of memory of the attacks after recovery.[12] Jean de Sponde believed that lycanthropy can be caused by noxious herbs which can drive man mad and affect his judgment and reason. He felt, however, that the devil will employ potions and unguents that have no power within themselves to affect the metamorphosis of man into wolf.[13] This position was also held by Sieur de Beauvoys de Chauvincourt, who subscribed to the belief that drugs and toxic substances were involved to help the devil create a spell, deceiving both the sorcerer and those who saw him.[14] In other words, under the influence of drugs, a person may hallucinate werewolves or see himself as a werewolf. Jean de Nynauld and Giovanni Battista Porta also implicated drugs and poisons in the causation of lycanthropy. Amongst the drugs and plants mentioned are cohoba, a noxious herb from Haiti, belladonna, different nightshades, opium, hyoscyamine, peyote, hashish, strychnine, stramonium, mandrake, and henbane. In the twentieth century yet another explanation is offered by psychoanalysts who see lycanthropy as a proper vehicle for sexual, sadistic, cannibalistic and necrophilic instincts, split off from the ego on an animal level, and thereby immune from guilt.[17]

The balance between these two different interpretations, religious-superstitious *versus* medical, has frequently been dominated by the first one, especially in Europe in the late Middle Ages and the sixteenth and seventeenth centuries, when lycanthropy was widespread and sometimes epidemic. With the prevalent religious belief that the disorder was a brand of sorcery and evidence of a pact with the devil, thousands of people were executed as werewolves. Despite these executions, the medical profession, as indicated above, increasingly emphasized the disease aspect and therefore treatment or incarceration into mental institutions occurred.

The clinical picture of the lycanthropes show an amazing consistency as ". . . pale, their vision is feeble, their eyes dry, tongue very dry, and the flow of saliva is stopped, but they are thirsty and their legs have incurable ulcerations from frequent falls".[7,8] The treatment included exorcism as well as the traditional treatment for patients suffering from melancholia, which used to be a broad diagnostic term. This treatment began with bloodletting to the point of fainting, whereupon the patient was treated with a wholesome diet and baths. He was subsequently purged with colocynth, dodder of thyme, aloe, wormwood, acrid vinegar, and quills. In chronic cases, vomiting was induced with hellebore.

The patient also obtained sedatives and his nostrils were rubbed with opium.[7,8]

Case 1

Mr. H., a 20-year-old single, unemployed white male from Appalachia, was admitted with a history of long and chronic drug abuse, including marijuana, amphetamines, psilocybin and LSD. His present sickness was precipitated by LSD and strychnine taken while he was in Europe with the United States Army ten months previously. He was out in the woods while he ingested the LSD, and felt himself slowly turning into a werewolf, seeing fur growing on his hands and feeling it grow on his face. He experienced a sudden uncontrollable urge to chase and devour live rabbits. He also felt that he had obtained horrible insight into the devil's world. After having been in this condition for two days, he rejoined his Army post but remained convinced that he was a werewolf. Looking for clues, he believed that the mess hall sign "feeding time" proved that other people knew that he was a wolf. He was sent to a psychiatrist who treated him with chlorpromazine† for a few months. Six months thereafter he was returned to the United States on medical evacuation status to a drug program, where he was observed for a few weeks with a diagnosis of "drug abuse-amphetamines". During the next few months, the patient quit all drugs except marijuana, but continued to be preoccupied with the werewolf transformation. He felt worse after he saw the movie "The Exorcist" two weeks prior to admission.

The background history reveals that the patient's father left home during Mr. H.'s infancy and denied his paternity of the patient, but not that of his two older brothers. The patient felt that the father did this to maintain credibility with his mistress, whom he subsequently married. His first step-father with whom he was very close, died in his presence, when he was seven. He lost his second stepfather through divorce in his early teens. The patient was very

---

†Thorazine

close to his mother. There is a family history suggestive of mental disease, and an older brother and a maternal cousin were denied admission to the Army because they were "weird and nervous".

The patient was sociable as a child. He started experimenting with hallucinogenic drugs in junior high. While in high school, he became interested in the occult and identified with a male priest who claimed to be a satanist. After high school the patient joined the Army where his drug use was intensified. Following his discharge from the Army after fourteen months he returned home and has been restless, hostile, agitated, anhedonic, socially withdrawn, and unable to maintain steady work. His complaints increased after his mother was notified that she would require a nephrectomy.

On admission the patient presented as a tense and suspicious young man who felt that the staff members might be possessed by or be tools of the devil. He had paranoid delusions, feeling that the devil at the end of each performance of "The Exorcist" goes out of the screen and possesses one of the movie goers. He had auditory hallucinations, hearing his thoughts aloud or his name being called, as well as visual hallucinations, during which he saw goats and black mass paraphernalia on the floor. When he looked in a mirror he occasionally saw a devil's claw over his eyes. He also believed that his thoughts were broadcast, and that the devil inserted thoughts into his mind and enabled him to read minds. He had unusual powers and felt that he could stare down dogs with his demoniacal gaze. He felt that the doctors put drugs in the patients' food to make them crazy. He showed marked ambivalence, seeking out doctors for long conversations, while at the same time expressing his fear of them. His affect was inappropriate and he would appear angry for no obvious reason, or giggle while discussing his stepfather's sudden death. There were somatizations of his delusion, and he attributed a shooting pain from the neck through the arms as a sign of possession. The patient gave a history of heavy and multiple drug use including LSD, amphetamines, mescaline, psilocybin, heroin and marijuana until his bad trip ten months ago, when he stopped taking LSD but continued to take amphetamines and marijuana. Since his discharge from the Army he continues to smoke marijuana regularly but has not taken any other drugs.

The MMPI was interpreted as ". . . compatible with an acute schizophrenic or toxic psychosis characterized by anxiety, obsessional thinking, agitation, religious delusions as well as bizarre sexual preoccupations and fears regarding homosexuality. Delusions of grandeur, ideas of reference and hallucinations may be present. A delusional system involving omnipotence, genius and special abilities may be present that could also be compatible with the profile of a male hysteric who has decompensated into a psychotic reaction."

The patient was treated with trifluo perazine†† and showed gradual improvement. At the time of his discharge thirty-two days after admission, he had dropped the belief that he was a werewolf or that he was possessed and, displayed no other overt psychotic determinants.

The patient was referred to an outpatient clinic near his hometown, two hundred miles from this hospital. He was seen for an interview at that clinic two weeks after his discharge and appeared polite but guarded, was preoccupied with satanism and had stopped his medications because they made him feel uneasy. No further contact was established with this patient, and it was thought by the staff that he perhaps felt threatened by the clinic. Attempts to call him for further visits failed.

Case II

Mr. W. is a 37-year-old single male farmer from Appalachia. At the time of his service in the United States Navy he had a normal and average IQ. Since his discharge after four years of service he has progressively and insidiously failed to function both as a farmer and in his daily activities. He has episodically behaved in a bizarre fashion, allowing his facial hair to grow, pretending that it was fur, sleeping in cemeteries and occasionally lying down on the highway in front of oncoming

††Stelazine

vehicles. There is also a history of the patient howling at the moon. Following two of these occasions, he was admitted to a psychiatric hospital. On the first admission he was given a diagnosis of "psychosis with mental deficiency", and marked deterioration of higher cortical functions was noted. During his second hospitalization, he was diagnosed as suffering from chronic undifferentiated schizophrenia, based on his bizarre behaviour since delusions or hallucinations could not be elicited while he was in hospital. During his third hospitalization, one year after his second hospitalization, the patient explained his bizarre behaviour by saying that he was transformed into a werewolf. The mental status examination showed a patient who was tidy yet dirty and sat in a slumped position. His facial expression was blank and he showed paucity of motor activity. He did not display any concern about his hospitalization and his affect was flat. His speech was slow, but in general logical and coherent, with impoverished thought processes. Although little rapport could be established, the patient was in general cooperative and compliant. On cognitive function testing he showed markedly impaired attention and concentration. His ability to calculate was severely impaired, recent memory was moderately impaired, and remote memory was spotty. The ability to make objective judgments and to abstract was adequate. On physical examination, soft neurological signs were found, including bilateral hyporeflexia of the triceps, a slow second phase of both knee jerks and a thick speech with regarded flow. The remainder of the neurological examination was negative and the family history was noncontributory and negative for neuropsychiatric problems. The patient's symptoms began after he was discharged from the Navy.

The patient had a positive brain scan, static, in the region of the right frontal cortex. Skull X-rays showed a lucid area in the right frontal region. The cerebral arteriogram did not show a mass lesion in the brain. The pneumoencephalogram showed no evidence of dilation, but the third ventricle was somewhat atypical in appearance. No pathological changes could be identified.

Psychological testing showed ". . . a mental age on the Peabody Picture Vocabulary Test of eight years one month and ten years five months respectively, corresponding to an IQ score of 57 and 68. On the Shipley Hartford Scale his vocabulary mental age was eleven years, nine months, his abstract mental age was eight years, four months and his conceptual quotient was 70. There was a variation in the testing and his verbal functioning level was at best in a mild retardation range with an IQ between 52 and 67. Considering his figure drawings and the Shipley Hartford Conceptual Quotient his level of impairment was even greater, probably in the moderate mental retardation range with an IQ between 36 and 51 or lower. There seemed to be indication of brain damage. On a concrete level, his ability to comprehend was surprisingly almost adequate. He was not capable of any abstract reasoning and psychomotor retardation was pronounced. If care was taken to communicate with him, he could communicate on a simple concrete level."

Because of his bizarre behaviour and his increasing dementia at an early age, a brain biopsy was performed. It was noted that the subarachnoid space was quite enlarged. The neurosurgeon noted at the time of the operation that the gyri of the brain were quite small, whereas the sulci were large, suggesting a 'walnut' brain. On microscopic examination, the cortical tissue revealed an unusual degree of astrocytosis with areas of cortical degeneration. There was no evidence of senile plaques or neurofibrillary traglex. These findings were not compatible with Alzheimer's disease.

The patient was discharged with a diagnosis of chronic brain syndrome of undetermined etiology. His psychotic behaviour has been successfully controlled with thioridazine, hydrochloride 50 mgm b.i.d.,††† and no further episodes of lycanthropy have been reported since his discharge one year ago, but he continues to be inactive, seldom reads, and on his last visit to the Outpatient Clinic it was noted that he offers little spontaneous conversation. He appears quiet and childlike, answering most questions with "yes", "no", or "I don't

†††Mellaril

know", but he did not show any evidence of abnormal behaviour or psychosis.

COMMENTS

Lycanthropy, by its very definition, would appear to point to a severe type of depersonalization. Many medical treatises from the past have indeed suggested that it is a form of hysteria. The endemic occurrence of the disorder and its mystical superstitious content have been used as supporting arguments. Many contemporary psychiatrists, when faced with the description of the recorded cases of the sixteenth and seventeenth centuries, would undoubtedly focus on the severe withdrawal, bizarre behaviour and delusions, impaired impulse control, and habit deterioration to support a diagnosis of schizophrenia.

The two presented cases shared lycanthropy but had a different diagnosis. The first was complicated by the history of drug use but was diagnosed as paranoid schizophrenia, perhaps precipitated and facilitated by drugs. The second case represented a chronic brain syndrome with periodic psychotic flare-ups. The common denominator would appear to be an onset precipitated by changes in brain disease in the second. Depersonalization has of course been frequently described by contemporary hallucinogenic drug users. The occurrence of depersonalization in convulsive disorders has also been noted. Therefore, the authors propose that in both instances an altered state of consciousness existed. In the first case, this was brought on by LSD and strychnine and continued casual marijuana use. In the second it must be assumed that a chronic altered state of consciousness was caused by irreversible brain disease, although the periodicity of his psychosis, occurring during the full moon, remains unexplained on an organic level.

Concerning drugs as causative agents, it is interesting to note that opium has been mentioned in a dual capacity, namely as a drug which can cause lycanthropy as well as a drug for its treatment. Wormwood is described as a cerebral stimulant, which has been used in absynthe and continues to be used in vermouth. The nightshades contain belladonna. Mandrake is described as a narcotic herb which contains hyoscyamine, scopolamine, and atropine. Stramonium is found in Jimson weed which contains hyoscyamine as does henbane, which is a narcotic, and is poisonous to fowl—hence its name. Columbus, while in the Caribbean, discovered cohoba, a snuff which produced trances and visual hallucinations among the Indians. Peyote was discovered by the Spanish explorers in West America as a hallucinogenic. All these substances are known to produce altered states of consciousness characterized by perceptual distortions such as hallucinations and illusions and a loss of ego boundaries, in which the subject experiences transcendental, oceanic, mystical or universal feelings. During this stage, the subject is highly vulnerable to suggestions and manipulations. [18] One may assume that excessive purgation or vomiting, with subsequent changes in the electrolyte balance, may also produce an altered state of consciousness. The clinical description of the lycanthrope with "feeble vision, dry eyes, dry tongue, no flow of saliva and thirsty" certainly suggests the use of atropine or related substances.

It is very likely that amongst the lycanthropes of antiquity were some "trippers". As LSD and marijuana became epidemic in the 1960s (with the benefit of newspapers, television and radio coverage), it is probable that similar but smaller drug epidemics existed in the past. The epidemic argument used in favour of hysteria might also be used to argue for drug-induced lycanthropy. Some of the substances used then continue to be in use now, notably Jimson weed, peyote, marijuana and opium. Although lycanthropy has been described as a disease of the past, the senior author has occasionally heard of shape shifting into an animal form experienced by people under the influence of hallucinogenic drugs. These two cases signify the continued existence of lycanthropy as a symptom in contemporary psychiatry disorders.

REFERENCES

1. Aetius: *De Lycanthropia* by Marcellus Sidetes translated by Francis Adams "The Seven Books of Paulus Aegeneta", *Vol. 1*, pp. 389–390. London, 1844.
2. Altomaris, Donato Antonio: De lupina insania in *Omnia Opera Venetics*, 79, folio, 1574.
3. Arieti, Silvano: Ed. *American Handbook of Psychiatry, Vol. I*, p. 11, New York, Basic Books Inc., 1974.
4. Bodin, Jean: *De la Demonomania des Sorciers*, Chapter VI, "De la Lycanthropie", Paris, Chez Jacques, 1580.
5. Chauvincourt, Beauvoys de: *Discours de la lycanthropie ou de la transmutation des hommes en Loups*, Paris, Louvain, 1599.
6. Fodor, N.: "Lycanthropy as a Psychic Mechanism", *J. Am. Folklore*, 58, 310–316, 1945.

7. Hasting, J.: Ed. *Encyclopedia of Religion and Ethics*, New York, Charles Scribner's Sons, *8*. 206–220, 1916.
8. Herbert, Jennings Rose: "Lycanthropy", *Encyclopedia Britannica, XIV*, pp. 509–511, 1964.
9. Lawson, J.C.: *Modern Greek Folklore*, Cambridge, England, University Press, 1910.
10. Ludwig A.M.: Altered states of consciousness, *Arch. Gen. Psych., 15*, 225, 1966.
11. Nynauld, Jean de: *De la lycanthropie, Transformation et Extase des Sorciers*, Chapters II, VI, Paris, Louvain, 1615.
12. Ovid: *Metamorphozes, Book I*, 211–239, translated into English verse by Mr. Dryden, London, 1693.
13. Porta, Giovanni Battista: *De Medicis Experimentis*, English translation *Natural Magick in XX Bookes, VIII*, 2, 219–220, London folio, 1658.
14. Sennert, Daniel: Practice Medicina, Lib. 1, pars. II, cap. XVI, in *Omnia Venetics*, 1628.
15. Sponde, Jean de: "Commentary upon Homer", p. 137–140, folio, *Bastiliae*, 1583.
16. Summers, Montague: *The Werewolf*, New Hyde Park, New York University Books, 1966.
17. Thyreaus, Peter, S.J.: *De Spiritum Apparitionibus*, Col. Agrippinae, p. 111–136, 1594.
18. Vergil: *Ecologues VIII*, translated by J.W. Mackail, 1889.

7

A Case of Lycanthropy

HARVEY A. ROSENSTOCK, *M.D.*[1]
KENNETH R. VINCENT, *Ed.D.*[2]

Lycanthropy, a psychosis in which the patient has delusions of being a wild animal (usually a wolf), has been recorded since antiquity. The Book of Daniel describes King Nebuchadnezzar as suffering from depression that deteriorated over a seven-year period into a frank psychosis at which time he imagined himself a wolf. Among the first medical descriptions of lycanthropy were those of Paulus Aegineta during the later days of the Roman Empire.[1] In his description of the symptom complex, Aegineta made reference to Greek mythology in which Zeus turned King Lycon of Arcadia into a raging wolf. Thereafter, references to lycanthropy appeared in the ancient literature. Many medieval theologians envisioned lycanthropy as a consequence of the evil eye.[2]

Delusions of being a wolf or some other feared animal are universal and, although rare in the industrialized countries, still occur in China, India, Africa, and Central and South America.[3,4] The animals in the delusional transformation include leopards, lions, elephants, crocodiles, sharks, buffalo, eagles, and serpents.[3,4]

Not infrequently, bizarre and chaotic sexuality is expressed in a primitive way through the lycanthropic symptom complex. Patients whose

[1,2]Hauser Clinic, Houston, Texas.

internal fears exceed their coping mechanisms may externalize them via projection and constitute a serious threat to others. Throughout the ages, such individuals have been feared because of their tendencies to commit bestial acts and were therefore hunted and killed by the populace. Many of these individuals were paranoid schizophrenics.[2]

CASE REPORT

A 49-year-old married woman presented on an urgent basis for psychiatric evaluation because of delusions of being a wolf and "feeling like an animal with claws." She suffered from extreme apprehension and felt that she was no longer in control of her own fate; she said, "A voice was coming out of me." Throughout her 20-year marriage she experienced compulsive urges toward bestiality, lesbianism, and adultery.

The patient chronically ruminated and dreamed about wolves. One week before her admission, she acted on these ruminations for the first time. At a family gathering, she disrobed, assumed the female sexual posture of a wolf, and offered herself to her mother. This episode lasted for approximately 20 minutes The following night, after coitus with her husband, the patient suffered a 2-hour episode, during which time she growled, scratched and gnawed at the bed. She stated that the devil came into her body and she became an animal. Simultaneously, she experienced auditory hallucinations. There was no drug involvement or alcoholic intoxication.

Hospital Course

The patient was treated in a structured inpatient program. She was seen daily for individual psychotherapy and was placed on neuroleptic medication. During the first 3 weeks, she suffered relapses when she said such things as "I am a wolf of the night; I am a wolf woman of the day . . . I have claws, teeth, fangs, hair . . . and anguish is my prey at night . . . the gnashing and snarling of teeth . . . powerless is my cause, I am what I am and will always roam the earth long after death . . . I will continue to search for perfection and salvation."

She would peer into a mirror and become frightened because her eyes looked different: "One is frightened and the other is like the wolf—it was dark, deep, and full of evil, and full of revenge of the other eye. This creature of the dark wanted to kill." During these periods, she felt sexually aroused and tormented. She experienced strong homosexual urges, almost irresistible zoophilic drives, and masturbatory compulsions—culminating in the delusion of a wolflike metamorphosis. She would gaze into the mirror and see "the head of a wolf in place of a face on my own body—just a long-nosed wolf with teeth, groaning, snarling, growling . . . with fangs and claws, calling out 'I am the devil.'" Others around her noticed the unintelligible, animal-like noises she made.

By the fourth week she had stabilized considerably, reporting, "I went and looked into a mirror and the wolf eye was gone." There was only one other short-lived relapse, which responded to reassurance by experienced personnel. With the termination of that episode, which occurred on the night of a full moon, she wrote what she experienced: "I don't intend to give up my search for [what] I lack . . . in my present marriage . . . my search for such a hairy creature. I will haunt the graveyards . . . for a tall, dark man that I intend to find." She was discharged during the ninth week of hospitalization on neuroleptic medication.

Psychological Data

On the Wechsler Adult Intelligence Scale, the patient's performance showed normal intellect; the subscale configuration was devoid of behavioral correlates associated with organicity, as was the Bender Motor Gestalt Test. On the Holtzman Ink Blot Technique, the performance was indicative of an acutely psychotic schizophrenic with distorted body image and gross sexual preoccupation. The Lovinger Sentence Completion Blank was corroborative. The Minnesota Multiphasic Personality Inventory was interpreted as showing an acute schizophrenic reaction with evidence of obsessional thinking, marked feelings of inferiority, and excessive needs for attention and affection.

DISCUSSION

We believed that the patient suffered from chronic pseudoneurotic schizophrenia. What is of particular interest is that the delusional material was organized about a lycanthropic matrix. Her symptom complex included the following classic symptoms:

1. Delusions of werewolf transformation under extreme stress.
2. Preoccupation with religious phenomenology, including feeling victimized by the evil eye.
3. Reference to obsessive need to frequent graveyards and woods.
4. Primitive expression of aggressive and sexual urges in the form of bestiality.
5. Physiological concomitants of acute anxiety.

These symptoms occurred significantly in the absence of exposure to toxic substances. Furthermore, the patient responded to the treatment protocol used for acute schizophrenic psychosis. After reviewing ancient and modern literature, it is felt that the differential diagnosis for lycanthropy should include consideration of all of the following possibilities: 1) schizophrenia, 2) organic brain syndrome with psychosis, 3) psychotic depressive reaction, 4) hysterical neurosis of the dissociative type, 5) manic-depressive psychosis, and 6) psychomotor epilepsy. The last item is mentioned because of reports that individuals suffering from lycanthropy have been described as being "prone to epilepsy" and suffering from intercurrent amnestic episodes.[3]

A search of modern literature* produced three cases. In two cases,[4] the patients were ultimately diagnosed as having paranoid schizophrenia, facilitated by involvement with hallucinogenic drugs, and chronic brain syndrome with periodic psychoses. In the third case, described by Morel in 1852, it seems that the patient suffered from a deteriorating psychotic depression.[5]

We believe that the metamorphosis undergone by the patient we have described provided temporary relief from an otherwise consuming sexual conflict that might have taken the form of a completed suicide.

Lycanthropy is a rare phenomenon, but it does exist. It should be regarded as a symptom complex and not a diagnostic entity. Furthermore, although it may generally be an expression of an underlying schizophrenic condition, at least five other differential diagnostic entities must be considered.

---

*Medlars II and Psychological Abstracts.

REFERENCES

1. Adams F: The Seven Books of Paulus Aegineta, vol 1. London, Sydenham Society, 1844, pp 389–390
2. Freedman AF, Kaplan HI, Sadock BJ: Comprehensive Textbook of Psychiatry, 2nd ed, vol 2. Baltimore, Williams & Wilkins Co. 1975, pp 13, 995, 1727
3. Summers M: The Werewolf. New York, University Books, 1966, pp 1–51
4. Surawicz F, Banta R: Lycanthropy revisited. Can Psychiatr Assoc J 20:537–542, 1975
5. Turke D: Dictionary of Psychological Medicine, vol 2. London, Morel, 1892, p 58

8

Another Case of Lycanthropy

PAULINE M. JACKSON, *M.D.*

SIR: I would like to add another example of lycanthropy to the case that was so well described by Harvey A. Rosenstock, M.D., and Kenneth R. Vincent, Ed.D. (Clinical and Research Reports, October 1977 issue).

I have a woman patient who gives a lifelong history compatible with schizoid personality traits but who first presented with a psychotic state at age 56. Her marriage had been deteriorating for several years, and immediately after an attempted reconciliation through sexual activity with her husband she believed that she had become a wild dog. When seen in the emergency room, she was making barking sounds, crouched down, cowering in the corner, extending her hands in claw-like fashion. During the intervals between the canine behavior she was very anxious and talked of being possessed by the devil. She was clearly quite frightened of other people at that time. Her dog-like behavior rapidly remitted with antipsychotic medication, but the next day she had many illusions and misidentified most strangers as friends and acquaintances. She was discharged after a short hospitalization and followed in supportive psychotherapy. At that time she refused to continue antipsychotic medication. She had erotomanic delusions that occupied increasingly more of her thoughts.

Five months after the first hospitalization she was admitted again,

---

Reprinted with permission from *American Journal of Psychiatry*, 1978, Vol. 135, 134–135.

this time having driven herself to the hospital in what appeared to be a fugue state. Again, her symptoms had developed after an attempt at sexual relationships with her husband. During that first night in the hospital she intermittently growled and clawed at the air while crouching on the floor, obviously in a panic. Two days later, she again developed a transient Capgras syndrome, this time in a negative sense, being convinced that I was an impostor and that I was making it impossible for the real Dr. Jackson to see her. She could remember nothing of the delusional material she had presented over the previous few weeks, insisting instead that she was happily married. By the next day (again, while on antipsychotic medication) she was relatively clear, identified people appropriately, and could describe the activities immediately before her admission, especially "turning into a wild dog."

She has now been out of the hospital for 8 months and is still receiving antipsychotic medication as well as psychotherapy. She often talks of her fear that she will turn into a wild dog again, and she tries to prevent this by avoiding sexual contact with her husband. Much as in the case reported by Drs. Rosenstock and Vincent, this patient's underlying psychodynamics include problems with the expression of aggression and sexual feelings, with considerable guilt and belief that sexual activity is subhuman.

9

Lycanthropy Lives On

PATRICK G. COLL
MB, FRCP(C)[1]
GERALDINE O'SULLIVAN
MB, BCh, BAO[2]
PATRICK A. BROWNE
LRCP, SI, MRCPsych[3]

Lycanthropy is the delusion in which an individual believes he has been transformed into an animal, traditionally a wolf. Descriptions of this syndrome are found in the earliest medical writings such as those of the Greek Paulus Aegineta in the seventh century A.D. (Adams, 1844). There is also a biblical description of the syndrome in the Book of Daniel. Nebuchadnezzar (605–562 B.C.), the king who rebuilt Babylon, succumbed to a lycanthropic state after suffering from an apparent depressive illness for seven years. St. Patrick is reported to have transformed Veneticus, King of Gallia, into a wolf (Arieti, 1974).

This syndrome gave rise to the folk belief in "werewolves" or sanguinary man-animals, who were said to change into their animal state under the influence of the full moon. (Summers, 1966). Community fear of such people attacking and eating human victims led to persecution in medieval Europe. This was institutionalised by ecclesiastical courts during the period of the Inquisition. (Lessa, 1967).

[1,2,3]Cork Regional Hospital, Wilton, Cork, Eire.

Reprinted with permission from *British Journal of Psychiatry,* 1975, Vol. 147, 201–202.

Delusions of animal metamorphosis are universal, and are more common in non-industrialised countries. Animals cited in delusional transformation, such as lions, tigers, hyenas, sharks, crocodiles and others, are reported from China, India, Africa, Central and South America. (Summers, 1966; Lessa, 1967). Whitigo psychosis among the native Indians of North America is a related syndrome. In this condition, the patient believes he has become a Whitigo, a legendary giant cannibalistic figure, and may progress to homicide and cannibalism. (Friedman *et al*, 1977). It is speculated that the rarity of the syndrome in Europe now is due partly to the virtual extinction of wolves in Europe.

Apart from historic descriptions, there have been at least four cases described in the medical literature over the past 10 years. (Surawitz & Banta, 1975; Rosenstock & Vincent, 1977; Jackson, 1978). We report here on a further case.

CASE HISTORY

Mrs. G. B. was a 66 year-old widow living with an unrelated family who were longtime friends of hers. She presented at our Unit with a seven-day history of disturbed behaviour. She had become aggressive towards some members of the family for no apparent reason. This was associated on a number of occasions with animal-like behaviour, during which she would go down on her hands and knees and "bark like a dog". This usually occurred when she was alone with one member of the family. In the preceding two weeks she had expressed fears of being alone and had refused to leave the house, claiming that there was a plot against her. She also questioned the origin of various noises and displayed other paranoid symptoms.

On admission, she had full recollection of her animal-like behaviour and said she had thought she was a dog during these episodes. She attributed this to the influence of the Devil who, she feared, would descend and take control of her if she were left alone. She also admitted having auditory hallucinations, which she felt originated from "evil spirits in the other half of the world". Her mood was depressed. Her appetite had decreased, with associated weight loss, and she was sleeping poorly. She feared her body was diseased and expressed a death-wish but denied suicidal intent. She was fully orientated and her cognitive functions were intact.

PAST HISTORY

She had had three previous psychiatric admissions, the most recent six months previously when she had suffered a depressive illness and been treated with electroconvulsive therapy and antidepressant medication. Her two previous admissions, 13 years earlier, had been characterised by depressive symptoms and by paranoid and nihilistic delusions.

FAMILY HISTORY

The patient's sister and a maternal aunt had histories of psychiatric illness, but we have no information about their diagnoses.

PERSONAL AND SOCIAL HISTORY

The patient came from a large farming family of 11 children. Her mother died when she was 10 years old and she was subsequently fostered by her uncle and his wife, thereby being separated from her siblings. She left school at age 14 and emigrated to England at 21, where she did factory work for six years. Following her marriage at age 27 she returned to Ireland. She described her marriage as happy but she had no children: the infertility was never investigated. After the death of her husband, 6 years previously, she had lived alone until she had moved in with her friends following her recent hospital admission. Prior to this illness she had been a gregarious, houseproud lady who maintained a small circle of close friends.

HOSPITAL COURSE

The initial diagnostic impression was of a paranoid psychosis, and Mrs. G. B. was treated with large doses of phenothiazines during the first month of her hospital stay. She remained hostile and aggressive, occasionally striking other patients, but she did not exhibit animal-like behaviour in hospital.

The diagnosis was then considered to be a psychotic depression and she was given anti-depressant medication and finally a course of electroconvulsive therapy. This was accompanied by the disappearance of her hallucinations and delusions and her aggressive behaviour also. She was discharged on a maintenance dose of antidepressant medication.

DISCUSSION

Interpretations of this syndrome have advanced from religious-superstitious to medical models and more recently to psychodynamic interpretations. The case histories of Rosenstock and Vincent (1977) and Jackson (1978), where the syndrome was precipitated by sexual intercourse, certainly lend themselves to psychodynamic interpretation. Psychoanalysts see the syndrome as an expression of primitive *id* instincts being expressed literally on an animalistic level through a splitting mechanism, thereby avoiding guilt feelings. (Surawicz & Banta, 1975).

Surawicz and Banta's (1975) case histories illustrate the medical model, where drug abuse (case 1) and an organic brain syndrome (case 2) are implicated. Carl Jung (1954) used a case of lycanthropy he saw to illustrate the sensitivity of children to their parent's unconscious conflicts. His patient, a devoted mother, had three daughters who loved her very much. However, they used to dream of her as a witch or dangerous animal, which they could not understand. Years later the mother developed a lycanthropic syndrome in which she would crawl about on all fours, imitating the grunting of pigs, the barking of dogs and the growling of bears.

Lycanthropy is essentially a severe form of depersonalisation, and the differential diagnosis must therefore include schizophrenia, manic-depressive psychosis, hysterical neurosis, psychotic depression and organic brain syndromes. (Rosenstock & Vincent, 1977). However, the symptom has been described for over 2,000 years, and in this age of rapidly changing psychiatric taxonomy it must be one of the oldest in the history of psychiatry.

REFERENCES

Adams, F. (1844). *The Seven Books of Paulus Aegineta*, Vol. 1. London: Syndenham Society.

Arieti, S. (1974). *American Handbook of Psychiatry*, Vol. 3. New York: Basic Books.

Freedman, A. F., Kaplan, H. L. & Sadcock, B. J. (1975). *Comprehensive Textbook of Psychiatry*, 2nd ed. Vol. 1 & 2. Baltimore: Williams & Wilkins.

Jackson, P. M. (1978) Another case of lycanthropy. *American Journal of Psychiatry*, 135, 134–135.

Jung, C. G. (1954). *Collected Works*, Vol. 17. London: Routledge & Kegan Paul.

Lessa, W. A. (1967) Lycanthropy. In *Colliers Encyclopaedia*, Vol. 15. New York: Growell, Collier & Macmillan.

Rosenstock, H. A. & Vincent, K. R. (1977) A case of lycanthropy. *American Journal of Psychiatry*, 134, 1147–1149.

Summers, M. (1966). *The Werewolf.* New York: University Books.

Surawicz, Frida G. & Banta, R. (1975) Lycanthropy revisited. *Canadian Psychiatric Association Journal*, 20, 537–542.

10

Lycanthropy
Alive and Well in the Twentieth Century

PAUL E. KECK
HARRISON G. POPE
JAMES I. HUDSON
SUSAN L. McELROY,
AARON R. KULICK[1]

SYNOPSIS Lycanthropy, the belief that one has been transformed into an animal (or behaviour suggestive of such a belief), has been described by physicians and clerics since antiquity, but has received scant attention in the modern literature. Some have even thought the syndrome extinct. However, in a review of patients admitted to our centre since 1974, we identified twelve cases of lycanthropy, ranging in duration from one day to 13 years. The syndrome was generally associated with severe psychosis, but not with any specific diagnosis or neurological findings, or with any particular outcome. As a rare but colourful presentation of psychosis, lycanthropy appears to have survived into modern times.

---

[1]Authors affiliated with McLean Hospital, Belmont, MA, and Harvard Medical School, Boston, MA.

Reprinted with permission from *Psychological Medicine*, 1988, Vol. 18, 113–120.

INTRODUCTION

Lycanthropy is the belief that one has been transformed into an animal, or the display of animal-like behaviour suggesting such a belief. (Strictly speaking, 'lycanthropy' refers to transformation into a wolf, whereas the term 'therianthropy' describes transformation into animals in general. However, the term 'lycanthropy' has now come to embrace other species.) The syndrome has intrigued physicians and clerics from antiquity to the present. Biblical accounts refer to the Babylonian King Nebuchadnezzar (605–562 B.C.) who suffered from the delusion that he was an ox during an apparent depressive illness (Driver, 1912); Hollywood has recently dramatized the story of an adolescent who believed that he was a bird (Wharton, 1978).

Historians have traced the origins of lycanthropy to Greek mythology, in which Zeus transformed the devious Lycaon into a wolf in retribution for attempting to trick him into eating human flesh (Innes, 1955). However the Greeks, in turn, may have adopted the myth from more ancient Phoenician cults (Summers, 1966). The myth has proved flexible, however, as subsequent descriptions of lycanthropy have incorporated themes of vengeance and demonic influence. In Irish folklore St. Patrick was said to have transformed Venetius, King of Gallia, into a wolf for his transgressions. In the Middle Ages, reflecting the spirit of the Inquisition, lycanthropy was ascribed to the influence of Satan (Kaplan & Sadock, 1985).

The aetiology of lycanthropy—both as described in folklore and as described in actual individuals—became the subject of heated controversy during the sixteenth and seventeenth centuries, as fledgling efforts at scientific understanding of the syndrome clashed with religious ideology. Jean Fernel, a sixteenth-century French physician, believed that human beings could be transformed into werewolves by the forces of Evil (Zilboorg & Henry, 1941). Leloyer (1588), his contemporary, argued that while individuals could not actually become animals, demonic powers could influence an individual to behave like one (see Zilboorg & Henry, 1941). Daniel Sennert (1577–1637) reiterated the belief that lycanthropy was attributable to demonic possession (Sennert, 1654). Bodin, also writing in the sixteenth century, presented an extensive review of lycanthropy in several editions of his work (Bodin, 1581, 1592, 1593). Bodin reported the cases of Garnier, Burgot and Verdun, three men in France who confessed to having turned into wolves and having eaten parts of nine children (Bodin, 1593). He also described lycanthropes from Constantinople, Germany, Greece, Asia and Egypt. In the suburbs of Cairo, for example, men reportedly transformed themselves into asses (Bodin, 1593). Bodin also believed that lycanthropy was entirely a supernatural phenomenon. He ridiculed the countervailing theory that lycanthropy could be attributable to a medical condition:

> Now if we admit that men have the power to cause roses to grow on a cherry tree . . . to change iron into steel or the form of silver into gold . . . how could one consider it strange if Satan were capable of changing one body to another, considering the vast power which God gave him? (Bodin, 1593)

Peter Thyreus took a more diplomatic but ambiguous position, postulating three distinct means of metamorphosis: one by hallucination, but two others by satanic influence (Thyreus, 1603).

However, other sixteenth-century physicians, such as Weyer (Zilboorg & Henry, 1941), Altomari (Surawicz & Banta, 1975), and Scot (Scot, 1886) focused on actual cases of lycanthropy rather than mythological accounts or accounts from folklore, and hence attempted to divorce lycanthropy entirely from theological-interpretation, postulating that the syndrome was the product of a disease state. The view was hardly novel: over a thousand years earlier, the Greek physician Paulus Aegineta had classified lycanthropy as a form of melancholia and suggested bloodletting as an effective treatment (Adams, 1864).

Yet, in spite of these latter opinions, lycanthropes were often tried, convicted and burned alive as demonically possessed (Bodin, 1593). Outbreaks of apparent mass hysteria or 'collective psychoses' occurred, resulting, in one instance, in the execution of 600 people suffering lycanthropic syndromes in France during the Middle Ages (Arieti, 1974). In another case of apparent hysterical lycanthropy in 1700, a group of nuns in a French convent were said to mew and behave as if transformed into cats (Arieti, 1974). Even in a culture as remote as that of nineteenth-century Japan, similar cases were described (Shinkichi, 1879).

Psychodynamic interpretations parallel, to some extent, the theological ascription of lycanthropy to the influence of evil, by regarding the syndrome as the product of split-off and unacceptable sexual and aggressive urges within an individual (Surawicz & Banta, 1975; Arieti, 1974; Rosenstock & Vincent, 1977; Jackson, 1978). Jung described a case of lycanthropy in which two daughters repeatedly dreamed of their mother transformed into an animal (Jung, 1954). Jung postulated that when, years later, the mother actually developed lycanthropy during a psychotic episode, her decompensation reflected the emergence of long-repressed primitive drives, recognized earlier in the unconscious of her daughters.

To our knowledge, only four reports, presenting five cases of lycanthropy, have appeared in recent years (Surawicz & Banta, 1975; Rosenstock & Vincent, 1977; Jackson, 1978; Coll *et al.* 1985). These are summarized in Table 1.

Experience at our centre over the last few years has suggested that lycanthropy may be more common than is suggested by the limited recent literature. Accordingly, we undertook a survey of cases observed within the last twelve years at McLean Hospital, a 250-bed private hospital in suburban Boston, Massachusetts, both to obtain further descriptions of the syndrome and to assess whether it was associated with psychiatric diagnosis, severity of illness, or outcome. We present below twelve cases of lycanthropy, representing, to our knowledge, the largest series to appear in the modern scientific literature.

TABLE 1.
Modern Reports of Lycanthropy

REPORT	PATIENT		DIAGNOSIS (BY AUTHOR)	LYCANTHROPIC DELUSION	OUTCOME
	AGE	SEX			
Surawicz & Banta (1975)	20	M	Paranoid schizophrenia; mixed substance abuse	Wolf	Remission with neuroleptic
	37	M	Chronic brain syndrome	Wolf	Remission with neuroleptic
Rosenstock & Vincent (1977)	49	F	Pseudoneurotic schizophrenia	Wolf	Remission with neuroleptic
Jackson (1978)	56	F	Schizoid personality traits	Dog	Remission with neuroleptic
Coll *et al.* (1985)	66	F	Delusional depression	Dog	Remission with neuroleptics, ECT, antidepressant

METHODS

Diagnostic Criteria

We began by choosing an operational definition for the diagnosis of lycanthropy. To do this, we analysed modern reports (Surawicz & Banta, 1975; Rosenstock & Vincent, 1977; Jackson, 1978; Coll *et al.* 1985) and drafted a definition that appeared to reflect a consensus of the various authors.

We designed the definition for use in both prospective and retrospective ascertainment of cases. Clearly, the belief that one has been transformed into an animal is central to the definition of lycanthropy. However, in our analysis we wanted to allow for circumstances in which a patient had displayed an array of behaviour (e.g. barking, howling, crawling on all fours, etc.) suggestive of an animal, but in which a patient did not explicitly announce that he or she was a particular type of animal. Therefore, we selected the following operational definition to include at least one of the following: (1) The individual reported verbally, during intervals of lucidity or retrospectively, that he or she was a particular animal. (2) The individual behaved in a manner reminiscent of a particular animal, i.e. howling, growling, crawling on all fours.

Survey Technique

Having established these criteria, we then contacted all members of the McLean Hospital attending staff, together with residents and nurses, and asked them to recall patients who had exhibited lycanthropy. This survey produced thirteen 'leads' which, upon review, yielded twelve cases meeting our criteria. We excluded one patient who was observed to have a 'cat-like' gait but who did not believe himself to be a cat and exhibited no other behaviour reminiscent of a cat or other animal.

In the remaining twelve cases we recorded available data from the chart and interviewed at least one physician who had examined the patient at the time of the putative episode of lycanthropy. We recorded from the chart the patients' ages, sex, psychiatric diagnosis, findings from neurological and physical examinations, routine laboratory data, EEG results, brain CT scan findings, detailed descriptions of the onset, nature and duration of lycanthropic behaviour, treatment and outcome.

Diagnoses were those made by the administrative ward psychiatrist according to the criteria of DSM-III (earlier DSM-II diagnoses were converted to DSM-III nosology on the basis of the extensive historical and observational data available in the chart). In five cases (cases 4–7 and 9) we also interviewed one or more members of the nursing staff who had witnessed the behaviour. We examined personally four of the patients (cases 7–10) during their actual episodes, and interviewed three other patients (cases 1, 4 and 5) one day to three weeks after their episodes had occurred.

RESULTS

The clinical features of the twelve patients are summarized in Table 2. Lycanthropy occurred in the context of an acute or chronic psychosis in 11 cases. Eight patients met DSM-III criteria for bipolar disorder (six were manic and two were depressed at the time of the index episode); two patients had schizophrenia; one patient had borderline personality disorder; and one patient, experiencing the chronic delusion that he was a cat, received the diagnosis of atypical psychosis, although he had experienced recurrent episodes of major depression in the past. One patient growled and contended that he was a Bengal tiger, and another patient, whose mania was resolving, said that he was a rabbit and hopped about the ward for a day. However, in these latter two cases the patients admitted that such behaviour was under their voluntary control. Each also admitted that he did not hold firmly to the belief that he was an animal. Thus, both of these patients met DSM-III criteria for factitious disorder with psychological symptoms (American Psychiatric Association, 1980) in addition to their other psychiatric diagnoses. Finally, one of the manic patients developed lycanthropy only after smoking hashish during the manic episode.

Although eight of 12 patients met DSM-III criteria for bipolar disorder when exhibiting lycanthropic behaviour, this observation should not be considered to show a specific association between lycanthropy and bipolar disorder for two reasons. First, nearly half of the patients with psychotic symptoms at our centre met DSM-III criteria for bipolar disorder, so that a finding of eight bipolar cases among a total of 12 cases might well be expected by chance. Secondly, two of the eight patients with a primary diagnosis of bipolar disorder experienced lycanthropic

TABLE 2.
Summary of Twelve Cases of Lycanthropy

CASE	AGE	SEX	DIAGNOSIS (DSM-III)	LYCANTHROPIC BEHAVIOUR	DURATION OF LYCANTHROPY	TREATMENT	OUTCOME	NEUROLOGICAL EXAMINATION	EEG
1	18	M	Bipolar disorder, manic; cannabis intoxication	Wolf: howling, crawling, barking, scratching (as if flea-infested)	3 weeks	Neuroleptic, lithium carbonate	Remission	Normal	Normal
2	38	M	Bipolar disorder, depressed	Gerbil: crawling, sleeping under bed, twitching face, startle responses	3 days	Neuroleptic, tricyclic antidepressant	Remission	Normal	
3	31	M	Schizophrenia	Unspecified: crawling, howling, hooting, clawing, stamping, defaecating in room	2 weeks	Neuroleptic	Treatment refractory	Peripheral neuropathy	1 left temporal spike/wave; 2 normal; 3 diffuse slowing
4	17	M	Bipolar disorder, manic; obsessive compulsive disorder	Dog: crawling, howling, barking, biting	2 weeks	Neuroleptic	Remission	Normal	Normal
5	16	M	Bipolar disorder, manic (rapid cycling); obsessive compulsive disorder	Unspecified: crawling, growling, barking, lordotic posturing	1 day	Neuroleptic	Partial remission	Normal	Normal
6	26	F	Bipolar disorder, manic	Bird: chirping, perching, head	7 days	Neuroleptic, lithium carbonate	Remission	Temporal pallor, right optic disc	1 normal; 1 generalized

7	37	F	Bipolar disorder, depressed	Cat: crawling, hissing, lordotic posturing, startle responses	1 day	Neuroleptic, tricyclic antidepressant	Remission	Normal	
8	24	M	Major depression, recurrent; atypical psychosis; alcohol abuse, in remission	Cat: crawling, mewing, hissing; hunting rodents and sexual activity with cats	13 years	Neuroleptic, tricyclic antidepressants, carbamazepine	Treatment refractory	Normal	Rare sharp wave activity right temporal area
9	29	M	Bipolar disorder, manic	Dog: crawling, howling, barking, hunching in corner	2 days	Neuroleptic	Remission	Normal	Normal
10	19	M	Schizophrenia	Wolf: howling, barking, sequestering food, assuming multiple feral postures	7 days	Neuroleptic	Partial remission	Normal	Normal
11	23	M	Bipolar disorder, manic; factitious disorder with psychological features	Rabbit: hopping	1 day	Neuroleptic, lithium	Remission	Normal	
12	28	M	Borderline personality disorder; factitious disorder with psychological features	Tiger: growling	1 day	None	Partial remission	Normal	Normal

symptoms which could not be directly attributed to their affective illness: as noted, one manic patient exhibited lycanthropy only after smoking hashish, and the other manic patient's lycanthropy appeared factitious. Thus, the distribution of diagnoses in the 12 patients was probably not significantly different from that of the hospital population as a whole.

In ten cases the patients identified themselves as specific animals; in two they exhibited feral behaviour sufficient to meet criterion (2) of our definition. In six cases lycanthropic behaviour remitted within one week of anti-psychotic drug treatment; in three other cases it abated within two to three weeks of treatment. In the two cases of factitious lycanthropy, symptoms resolved following confrontation. However, patient 8 continues to suffer from the delusion that he is a cat despite treatment with adequate trials of anti-psychotics, tricyclic antidepressants and carbamazepine, as well as ongoing insight-orientated psychotherapy. Of the patients with non-factitious lycanthropy, six apparently believed themselves to be, or acted like, wolves or dogs; two believed themselves to be cats; one patient believed himself a gerbil (he had raised gerbils as a hobby for six years); and one, a bird. It is interesting to speculate that the species of animal chosen may have specific psychological implications in individual cases. However, lacking detailed anamnestic material on the individual cases, such speculations are beyond the scope of this report.

No patients had significant medical illness or metabolic abnormalities as determined by physical examination by an internist and by routine laboratory data. Of the nine patients who received EEGs, two had non-specific abnormalities; one other patient had an EEG which revealed a left temporal lobe spike and wave pattern, but this was not replicated on five subsequent EEGs. The remaining six patients had normal waking EEGs. Two patients had minor neurological abnormalities (mild peripheral neuropathy; temporal field pallor on the disc of the right retina). All others had normal neurological examinations. On the recommendation of neurology consultants, only two patients received CT scans of the brain; one was normal and one showed nonspecific abnormalities (Table 2).

The presence of lycanthropy had no apparent relation to prognosis. Seven of the eight patients with bipolar disorder recovered completely from their manic or depressive episodes; the seventh displayed a partial remission. One schizophrenic patient had a reduction in the severity of his thought disorder and auditory hallucinations, together with a remission of his lycanthropic delusions, but remained residually psychotic. The other schizophrenic patient showed little response to treatment, although his lycanthropic delusions remitted. The patient with borderline personality disorder displayed a prompt remission of his lycanthropic behaviour, but only modest short-term improvement in his other symptoms. As previously noted, one patient has maintained the fixed delusion that he is a cat. We describe this case briefly below.

CASE 8

A 24-year-old single male presented to McLean Hospital with a history of recurrent major depression, a brief period of alcohol abuse, and the belief that he was a cat trapped inside a human body. This belief has persisted, without interruption, for 13 years.

The patient stated that he had known that he was a cat since this secret was imparted to him by the family cat, who subsequently taught him 'cat language'. Though gainfully employed, the patient continued to spend virtually all of his spare time in feline activities. He lived with cats, had sexual activity with them, hunted with them, and frequented cat night spots in preference to their human equivalents. His greatest—but unrequited—love was for a tigress in a local zoo. He hoped one day to release her.

The patient's lycanthropic delusions remained refractory to treatment with haloperidol, tricyclic antidepressants, carbamazepine, and six years of insight-oriented psychotherapy.

DISCUSSION

Though accounts of lycanthropy can be traced back to ancient times, modern descriptions of the syndrome are limited to four reports, describing five patients (Surawicz & Banta, 1975; Rosenstock & Vincent, 1977; Jackson, 1978; Coll *et al.* 1985). Indeed, a recent textbook of psychiatry (Arieti, 1974) describes the syndrome as extinct, and lycanthropy does not appear in the American Psychiatric Association's *Psychiatric Glossary* (Werner *et al.* 1984). However, our survey produced 12 cases of lycanthropy among approximately 5000 psychotic patients treated at McLean Hospital within the last 12 years. These observations suggest that lycanthropy, though unusual, is very much alive in the twentieth century.

Given that the series was small, and that not all patients were examined personally by the authors, our conclusions must remain tentative. However, several impressions emerge. First, lycanthropy does not appear specific to any particular disorder; it was observed in mania, depression, schizophrenia, atypical psychosis, cannabis intoxication superimposed on mania, and factitious disorder with psychological symptoms. Nor does lycanthropy appear to be associated with any particular neurological abnormalities: neurological examination, EEG and brain CT scan findings in our patients were unremarkable. Rather, lycanthropy appears to be a non-specific sign or symptom occasionally seen in severe functional psychosis or, less commonly, as a factitious psychological symptom.

Phenomenologically, the majority of our cases resemble those described in psychotic persons in earlier centuries. The two cases of factitious lycanthropy bear a similarity to medieval cases in which lycanthropy appeared as a form of mass hysteria. In these latter cases lycanthropic behaviour was probably under voluntary control and perhaps fulfilled unconscious or conscious fantasies for those afflicted.

Prognostically, lycanthropy does not appear to represent an ominous sign: seven of the 12 patients experienced a complete remission of their primary disorder, three had a partial remission, and two have remained, thus far, unresponsive to treatment. The apparent lack of association between lycanthropy and outcome is consistent with other studies, which have suggested that the depth of psychosis does not predict prognosis (Pope & Lipinski, 1978).

In summary, like other curious and memorable syndromes, such as those of Capgras and de Clerambault, lycanthropy persists as an occasional but colourful feature of severe, and occasionally factitious, psychosis. However, it appears that the delusion of being transformed into an animal may bode no more ill than any other delusion.

REFERENCES

Adams, F. (1864). *The Seven Books of Paulus Aegineta*, Vol. 1. Sydenham Society: London.

Arieti, S. (1974). *American Handbook of Psychiatry*, Vol. 3, pp. 719–770. Basic Books: New York.

Bodin, I. (1581). *Andegavenis de Magorum Daemonomania*, Vol. 4. Thoman Guarinum: Basile.

Bodin, I. (1592). *Demonomania de gli Stregoni, cioe, Furori, et Malie de Demoni*, Vol. 3. Presso Aldo: Venice.

Bodin, I. (1593). *De la Demonomanie des Sorciers.* Chez Iehan Keerberghe: Anvers.

Coll, P. G., O'Sullivan, G. & Browne, P. J. (1985). Lycanthropy lives on. *British Journal of Psychiatry* 147, 201–202.

Driver, S. R. (1912). The Book of Daniel. *Cambridge Bible for Schools and Colleges.* Cambridge University Press: Cambridge.

Innes, M. M. (1955). *The Metamorphoses of Ovid.* Penguin: Harmondsworth.

Jackson, P. M. (1978). Another case of lycanthropy. *American Journal of Psychiatry* 135, 134–135.

Jung, C. G. (1954). *Collected Works*, Vol. 17. Routledge & Kegan Paul: London.

Kaplan, H. L. & Sadock, B. J. (1985). *Comprehensive Textbook of Psychiatry* (third edn). Vols. 1 and 2. Williams & Wilkins: Baltimore.

Pope, H. G. & Lipinski, J. F. (1978). Diagnosis in schizophrenia and manic-depressive illness. A reassessment of the specificity of 'schizophrenic' symptoms in the light of current research. *Archives of General Psychiatry* 35, 811–828.

Rosenstock, H. A. & Vincent, K. R. (1977). A case of lycanthropy. *American Journal of Psychiatry* 134, 1147–1149.

Scot, R. (1886). *Discovery of Witchcraft*, Vol. 1. Clarendon Press: Oxford.

Sennert, D. (1654). *Practicae Medicinae de Capitis, Cerebri, et Sensuum Externorum Morbis & Symptomatibus.* Venice.

Shinkichi, T. (1879). Is lycanthropy confined to the Province of Shikohu? [transl.] *Tokei Ijishenshi* 86, 364–370.

Summers, M. (1966). *The Werewolf.* University Books: New York.

Surawicz, F. G. & Banta, R.(1975). Lycanthropy revisited. *Canadian Psychiatric Association Journal* 20, 537–542.

Thyreus, P. (1603). *De Obessis a Spiritibus Daemoniorum Hominibus.* Societatis iesu Doctore.

Werner, A., Campbell, R. J., Frazier, S. H., Stone, E. M. & Edgerton, J. (1984). *The American Psychiatric Association's Psychiatry Glossary.* American Psychiatric Press: Washington, D.C.

Wharton, W. (1978). *Birdy.* Alfred A. Knopf: New York.

Zilboorg, G. & Henry, G. W. (1941). *A History of Medical Psychology.* Norton: New York.

PART III

DEMONIACAL POSSESSION

Nihil á Spiritu, multa ficta, pauca á morbo.

("Nothing from the spirit, many things simulated, a few things from disease.")

Conclusion of the physicians of Paris in their report to the King of France regarding their investigation of the demoniac Marthe Brossier, *Discours veritable sur le faict de Marthe Brossier de Romorantin pretendue demoniaque* (Paris, 1599).

Introduction

"If wee want none other signes of the *divels* possession, but those set downe by the *Evangelists*, then every person that is Epileptike . . . every *Melancholike*, and every *Frantike* person shall have the *Devill* in their bodies, and there will be moe *Demoniakes* in the world, then there are *Fooles*."

Michel Marescot and the physicians of Paris,
A True Discourse . . . Translated out of French into English by Abraham Hartwell (London, 1599).

"The belief that one is possessed by another person, spirit, or entity may occur as a symptom of Multiple Personality Disorder. In such cases the complaint of being 'possessed' is actually the experience of the alternate personality's influence on the person's behavior and mood."

American Psychiatric Association,
Diagnostic and Statistical Manual of Mental Disorders, Third Edition, Revised, 1987.

POSSESSION: A WORLDWIDE PHENOMENON

One of the most ancient beliefs of humankind is that a spirit, force, or alien entity of some sort can enter a person's body and paralyze or supplant the will or volition of that person. These alien forces can be good or evil, invited or uninvited, and can either leave willingly or must be exorcised. By and large, when the possessing entity is uninvited, the psychological disruption in the sense of self and in behavior is generally considered harmful. This is why, for example, in many societies worldwide (nonliterate and so-called civilized), possession is considered a major factor in the cause of mental disease. Possession is also thought to be a major cause of many physical ailments as is suggested in the New Testament where the influence of possession by malevolent demons leads to paralysis, laming, and deafness.

There is a vast anthropological literature on cross-cultural beliefs in possession and on the behaviors and the observed altered states of consciousness that are interpreted as being due to alien entities or spirits possessing human beings. Perhaps the best single brief overview of the anthropological perspective can be found in the book *Possession* (1976) by anthropologist Erika Bourguignon of Ohio State University. Elsewhere, in a statistical study of possession beliefs and forms of institutional altered states of consciousness in 488 selected societies, Bourguignon (1973) found in her Cross-Cultural Study of Dissociational States conducted between 1963 and 1968 that fully 74 percent of them maintained some form of belief in spirit possession. Although not universal, such beliefs were clearly widespread, and with great regional differences. Furthermore, 52 percent of those world societies having a belief in possession also have some form of institutionalized "possession trance" (such as the *voudou* religion of Haiti). In these cases, usually during a ritual, certain selected individuals (often females) willfully become possessed by a particular deity or spirit for various socially sanctioned reasons. These institutionalized possession trances are thus not indigenously considered forms of mental illness. Bourguignon is emphatic on this anthropological distinction when she writes:

> Possession, as we have insisted, is a belief, a cultural belief, a shared and not an idiosyncratic belief. Insofar as the behavior involves acting out a personality which is believed in, concerning which there are shared expectations, to that extent surely "possession states" cannot exist in societies where such beliefs are absent. Nevertheless, if we speak in very general terms about dissociation, fugue states, multiple personalities, fainting, functional epileptic seizures and other behavior of an apparently hysterical type, then the behavior is probably universal and occurs in all societies; however, it should not properly be referred to as "possession states." (Bourguignon, 1976, 10)

The fact that for many centuries the medical profession in our culture has not officially recognized the reality of spirit possession as a cause of mental distress or physical illness is reflected in the passage above, and both are congruent with Bourguignon's anthropological distinction.

Perhaps the classic reference on the phenomenon of possession is the book *Obsession and Possession by Spirits Both Good and Evil, in Oriental and Occidental Spiritualism and Occultism, Among Primitive Races, In Antiquity, the Middle Ages, and Modern Times* by German philosopher and psychologist T. K. Oesterreich. It first appeared in German in 1921 and then later appeared in English in 1930 (D. Ibberson, translator). Oesterreich includes many citations from rare historical, anthropological, and psychiatric texts, many of which have never been translated into English. Oesterreich performed a useful service by distinguishing states of "spontaneous" possession from those of "voluntary" possession, the latter largely comprising the deliberately induced "possession trance" altered states of consciousness that Bourguignon studied. Oesterreich also presages current interest in the phenomenon of possession as a type of dissociative disorder, and is astute when remarking in his chapter on "The External Signs of Possession" that the "changes in countenance" match "the classic cases of double personality (*dédoublement de personnalité*)" in the works of French *aliénistes* Azam (*Hypnotisme, double conscience et altérations de la personnalité*, Paris, 1887) and Bourru et Burot (*Variations de la personnalité*, Paris, 1888).

Although Oesterreich spent considerable time documenting the evidence for voluntary possession, he provided no theory as to why individuals would actually seek out such experience in the first place. It was not until the 1940s that anthropologists began to examine the wider societal context of possession trance and began to observe that in most male-dominated cultures one of the few avenues to power and prestige within the community that women could take was to become involved in possession trance behaviors, largely within the context of ritual. As mediums or vessels through which the gods spoke, women could find ways to communicate needs and exert power to enact social changes. By the 1950s, when much of anthropology was still under the sway of the Freudian psychoanalytic tradition through "culture and personality" studies, more psychologically beneficial effects such as catharsis were posited as the positive goals of possession trance participation.

With Bourguignon's (1973; 1976) work, the study of spirit possession began to be viewed within the context of altered states of consciousness, and the phenomenology of possession trance was compared and contrasted with other types of altered states of consciousness that were also institutionalized within certain cultures. Prince (1968) likewise edited a collection of papers largely devoted to this perspective. British social anthropologist I. M. Lewis (1971) contributed what may be the last comprehensive treatment of spirit possession in his book *Ecstatic Religion: An Anthropological Study of Spirit Possession and Shamanism.* Although Lewis' writings (1971; 1986) and those of most others in the field generally discuss the phenomenon of spirit possession in terms of group dynamics, a volume edited by Crapanzano and Garrison (1977) presents ten detailed individual case studies of spirit possession from cultures around the world. Of particular interest to students of Western manifestations of spirit possession (spiritualism, Pentacostalism, the case of the possession and exorcism of German college student Anneliese Michel in the 1970s, etc.) are the works of anthropologist Felicitas Goodman (1974; 1981; 1988).

PSYCHIATRY: FROM DEMONS TO DISEASES

Persons suffering from various forms of mental distress often report the feeling of seemingly autonomous forces moving in them and through them but that are not moved by them. The idea that ego-alien thoughts, feelings, and behaviors may be due to the volitional action of personified forces or entities is as old as humankind and is quite commonly reported today, as the case histories in this section demonstrate. The belief that spirit intrusion causes mental and physical distress is still quite alive even in our own "civilized" culture.

Contrary to the claims of many of the early historians of psychiatry (e.g., Zilboorg, 1941), all mental disorders were not thought to be caused by demoniacal possession in classical, Medieval, and Renaissance Europe. Indeed, as Kemp (1990) and Kemp and Williams (1987) have persuasively documented, many mental disorders have always been believed to have a biological or a behavioral basis. The roots of biological psychiatry, therefore, are actually quite ancient.

However, throughout the centuries in Europe, especially by the 16th century, the range of disorders that was attributed to demoniacal possession gradually narrowed. Epilepsy in particular was finally generally recognized to be a physiological disorder rather than a supernatural one by the end of the 16th century. The classic work on the history of epilepsy and the evolution of its various supernatural and natural etiologies is that by Temkin (1945). Of particular interest is Temkin's (1945, p. 138) citation of the skeptical opinion of the 16th century physician Riolan (1538–1606), who asserted in cases of "enthusiasm" (possession by a deity) that, "It is not necessary for us to have recourse to a demon as the last point of refuge, since we have a natural cause." However, Riolan's "natural cause" was based on the antiphlogistic or humoral theory of disease, for he felt it was the effect of "melancholic vapors of phantasy" that caused the disorder.

The difficulties of differential diagnosis in 14th century Europe can be illustrated in the case history of Flemish painter Hugo van der Goes (1435?–1482). In 1480, five years after joining the monastic community of the Roode Clooster near Brussels, Hugo came down with a "strange disorder of his imagination." He screamed incessantly that he was "doomed" and condemned to eternal damnation. Attempts at self-mutilation and possibly suicide were prevented when his fellow monks physically restrained him. The chronicler of the Roode Clooster and its *infirmarius*, Gaspar Ofhuys (1456–1523) wrote of the medical controversy surrounding the case:

> certain people talked of a peculiar case of *frenesis magna*, the great frenzy of the brain. Others, however, believed him to be possessed of an evil spirit. There were, in fact, symptoms of both unfortunate diseases present in him, although I have always understood that throughout his illness he never once tried to harm anyone but himself. This, however, is not held to be typical of the frenzied or the possessed. In truth, what it really was that ailed him only God can tell. (cited in Rosen, 1968, p. 145)

A useful historical survey of cases of possession and exorcism in France and England in the late 16th and early 17th centuries is provided by historian D. P. Walker. In it, Walker (1981) analyzes the differential diagnosis options available to physicians of that era: "Faced with a case of supposed possession a sixteenth-century observer had the choice of three possible kinds of explanation: first, a supernatural cause, a devil; second, disease; third, fraud" (p. 15). As a historian, Walker argues that he cannot accept supernatural explanations for the cases of possession that he documents, so he attributes them largely to "disease" and to "fraud." In so doing, he agrees with the Royally commissioned skeptical physicians of Paris headed by Michael Marescot who examined the self-proclaimed demoniac Marthe Brossier (whose proclamations were feeding into the considerable political unrest between Catholics and Protestants at that time): "*nihil à spiritu, multa ficta, pauca à morbo.*"

Modern psychiatric and psychological interpretations of cases of possession have followed these same guidelines. If a true mental disorder is suspected, it is probably due to one of the dissociative disorders. Allegations of fraud range from outright deceit to explanations of possession and the efficacy of "exorcism" that are due to "role enactment" expectations as described by social role and social learning theory (Spanos & Gottlieb, 1979). The present mental disorder in *DSM-III-R* (1987) that the American Psychiatric Association observes may involve signs and symptoms most like the ancient cases of demoniacal possession—multiple personality disorder—has likewise been attributed by skeptics to outright fraud or otherwise accountable by social role theory (Aldridge-Morris, 1989) or other social-psychological factors (Kenny, 1986).

Around the year 1800, the first modern psychiatric texts being written by physicians ("lunatic-doctors," "mad-doctors," or "*aliénistes*") who worked in large institutions for the insane ("mad-houses" or "asylums") began to appear. The vestiges of ancient medicine were clear in descriptions of the treatment of the mentally ill throughout the early 19th century: for when Philippe Pinel (1806) claimed in his landmark *Traite médico-philosophique sur l'alientation mentale, ou la manie* of 1801 that the "usual system of treatment" was "bleeding, bathing and pumping" (p. 287), he was revealing that the ancient antiphlogistic or humoral theory of mental illness was still the rationale for treatment. According to the humoral theory, many mental illnesses were caused by an "excess" of one or more of the four humors, particularly an excess of "hot blood" that needed to be eliminated through venesection or leeching. What is of interest is that just as in the ancient medical manuals, the authors of these early psychiatric texts also felt that the issue of demoniacal possession and mental illness had to be addressed.

Pinel set the tone for later psychiatric authorities with his pointed dismissal of supernatural explanations for cases of purported demoniacal possession. In his 1801 classic, he writes:

> Can we suppose the demoniacs, whose histories are recorded in theological writings, to be any more than extravagant mani-

> acs? We need only to visit a lunatic asylum in order to appreciate justly the nature of their pretended inspiration. In a word, demoniacs of all descriptions are to be classed either with maniacs or melancholics. (pp. 237–238)

The second great French *aliéniste* of the early 19th century, J. E. D. Esquirol, considered the issue of possession to be of great enough importance to devote a chapter to the description of a mental disorder he called "demonomania" in his *Maladies Mentales* of 1838. In that chapter, Esquirol is blunt in his denial of supernatural causes for demoniacal possession: "I shall show farther on, that demoniacal possession is a true monomania" (Esquirol, 1845, p. 237). Although Pinel tended to rely upon ancient terms for his classification of mental disorders (e.g., mania, melancholy, frenzy), Esquirol renamed many disorders and came up with new concepts, including that of "monomania." According to psychiatric historian Goldstein (1987), whose chapter on monomania is the best historical sketch to be found on this disorder in English (pp. 152–196), monomania "denoted an idée fixe, a single pathological preoccupation in an otherwise sound mind." According to analyses of the records of French institutions in the first half of the 19th century, monomania was the most common diagnosis given to institutionalized mental patients. Cases of demonomania may have been subsumed under this broader diagnostic category.

Esquirol finds there are two types of demonomania and they depend on the nature of the purported possessing entity. If a person is possessed by angels or saints or is otherwise in communication with God, he or she is considered to have *theomania*. If the person is experiencing possession at the hands of a malevolent spirit, demon, or other entity, then the diagnosis is *cacodemonomania* (from the Greek for bad demon mania). Following Esquirol's suggestion, 20th century clinicians have borrowed the term *cacodemonomania* to refer to modern case reports of this phenomenon, as the case histories that are reproduced in this section attest.

Given the dissociative nature of two of the three topics of this book—lycanthropy and demoniacal possession—it is interesting to note that Esquirol likewise recognized a possible interrelationship. He writes: "Connected with demonomania as a sub-variety, is Zoanthropy; a deplorable aberration of the mind, which perverts the instinct even, and persuades the lypemaniac that he is changed into a brute"

(Esquirol, 1845, pp. 250–251). What Esquirol may have been attempting here is an early classification scheme for what we now call the dissociative disorders.

POLYPSYCHISM

Demoniacal possession was usually given at least cursory mention in psychiatric texts throughout the 19th and 20th centuries, all of which strictly denied a supernatural explanation for the disorder. However, near the end of the 19th century when the idea of an unconscious mind was widely discussed, philosophers and psychologists began to explore the disorders of consciousness found in mesmerism or in cases of double personality or hysteria and speculated on what such phenomena may mean for understanding the "normal" mind. As Ellenberger (1970) has noted, models of the mind based on *polypsychism* were widely discussed. Pierre Janet's classic *L'Automatisme Psychologique* (1889) provided a wealth of clinical material to support the phenomenon of separate streams of consciousness in parallel operation within the same individual, and it did much to establish the concept of *dissociation* in psychology. The essential idea of polypsychism was that a disunity of consciousness was not inconsistent with a unity of self, and that the human mind may be a multiplicity within a unity.

Since phenomena that did indeed resemble cases of demoniacal possession as reported by the ancients were still appearing, the theory that we all are comprised of "multiple selves" (James, 1890) or parts was advanced to eliminate reliance on a supernatural explanation, even though many of the proponents of such theories were open to the reality of such a spirit world. For example, William James studied spiritualistic mediums firsthand and in his classic *The Principles of Psychology* (1890) he argues, ". . . I am persuaded that a serious study of these trance-phenomena is one of the greatest needs of psychology, and I think that my personal confession may possibly draw a reader or two into a field which the *soidistant* 'scientist' usually refuses to explore" (p. 396). Elsewhere, in a letter from James to a colleague dated February 1, 1879, he tells of a lecture he is to give on "Demoniacal Possession" at the New York Academy of Medicine and confesses to his friend:

> I am not as positive as you are . . . in the belief that the obsessing agency is really demonic individuals. I am perfectly

> willing to adopt that theory if the facts lend themselves best to it, for who can trace the limits to the hierarchies of personal existence in the world? But the lower stages of automatism shade off so continuously into the highest supernormal manifestations, through the intermediary ones of imitative hysteria and 'suggestibility' that I feel as if no one *general* theory as yet would cover all the facts. So that the most I will plead for before the neurologists is the recognition of demon possession as a regular 'morbid-entity' whose commonest homologue is the 'spirit-control' observed in test mediumship, and which tends to become the more benign and less alarming, the less pessimistically it is regarded. This last remark seems certainly to be true. Of course I will ignore the sporadic cases of old fashioned malignant possessions which still occur today. I am convinced that we stand with all of these things at the threshold of a long enquiry, of which the end appears as yet to no one, least of all myself. (cited in Taylor, 1982, p. 109)

James then goes on in the letter to laud the work of F. W. H. Myers (1903) as the best and most comprehensive theoretical system to account for the phenomenon of possession and its relationship to polypsychism. Myers' theory of subliminal selves was considered a classic in its day, and is noted as influential by Ernest R. Hilgard in his important volume, *Divided Consciousness: Multiple Controls in Human Thought and Action* (1977/1986), although he largely discounts the metaphysical speculations in the second volume of Myers' work. Another important work of recent publication that supports the notion of the multiplicity of mind is that of Beahrs (1982).

In his famous phenomenological study, *Psychology From an Empirical Point of View* (1874/1973), which otherwise provides an excellent description of the multiplicity of mind, Franz Brentano seems to leave open the possibility of true demoniacal possession when he writes:

> First of all, when we teach the unity of consciousness, we do not maintain in any way that different groups of mental phenomena, which do not belong to one and the same reality, can never be connected with one and the same connected physical body. We find such a relation in corals where countless little animals appear to have a common bodily life in one and the

> same stem. The simultaneous mental phenomena of one little animal and another do not form a real unity. But there is also no inner perception which apprehends their simultaneous existence. Consequently, it would in no way run counter to our definition if there were another self besides me present within my body, as though my body were possessed by one of those evil spirits whose exorcisms are so frequently reported in the Scriptures. There would be no real unity between the consciousness of this spirit and my consciousness, but then I would not directly apprehend its mental phenomena along with my own, either. (Brentano, 1874/1973, p. 164)

However, in the footnote added by editor Oskar Kraus to a 1925 edition of Brentano's text, this passage is explained with the statement that, "Modern studies of so-called 'possession' and the so-called split personality confirm that all of the pertinent phenomena belong to the same substantive self" (Brentano, 1874/1973, p. 164). This succinct definition of the concept of polypsychism is directly applicable to phenomenological descriptions of the late 20th century diagnostic category that accounts for many reports of demoniacal possession—multiple personality disorder.

MULTIPLE PERSONALITY

The history of the concept of dissociation and of multiple personality disorder is competently covered in the collection of essays edited by Quen (1986) and need not be reviewed here. An especially good summary of the history of multiple personality disorder can be found in the textbook by NIMH researcher Frank Putnam (1989), presently considered the best in existence on the subject.

As noted previously, the similarities between cases of demoniacal possession and persons with double personality, alternating personalities, double conscience, double consciousness, or multiple personalities has long been noted. In his textbook on multiple personality disorder, Canadian MPD authority Colin Ross (1989) has a detailed section devoted to "The Evolution of Demon Possession into Multiple Personality Disorder" and suggests that we call modern manifestations of demoniacal possession by a new name: postdemonic demon possession.

> In the modern world, Christian religion no longer exists as the organizing principle or guiding core of most medical and therapeutic practice. Most psychotherapy is agnostic or atheistic. In professional journals and books there are no techniques, theories, or viewpoints it would make sense to call *spiritual.* Not surprisingly there is also no demon possession. In this cultural climate any alleged cases of demon possession can therefore be described as postdemonic, from the perspective of the mainstream. (Ross, 1989, p. 25)

Changes in facial expression, voice, identity, and behavior are reported manifestations that are common to both demoniacal possession and multiple personality—as is the subjective report by the afflicted persons of being possessed or sharing the same physical body with two or more identities. The official psychiatric position is that these alternate personalities are dissociated bits of consciousness that must be integrated with the "birth personality" to achieve personality unification. Further, it is posited that these streams of consciousness were split-off due to severe trauma early in life, and this led to the creation of autonomous alternate personalities. No supernatural explanations need be invoked.

However, there are some clinicians who have worked with MPD patients who claim that they cannot account for all of the alternate personalities based on the traumatic events of a person's life, and thus, incredibly, they actually entertain the possibility of actual possession by discarnate entities. California psychiatrist Ralph Allison, who was perhaps the first person to seriously push for the recognition of multiple personality disorder by psychiatry in the 1970s and who pioneered the psychotherapy of MPD, writes in his book *Minds in Many Pieces*, "The discovery of an entity who doesn't serve any recognizable purpose presents a diagnostic problem. Interestingly enough, such entities often refer to themselves as spirits. Over the years I've encountered too many such cases to dismiss the possibility of spirit possession completely" (Allison, 1980, p. 184). Swiss psychiatrist Hans Naegeli-Osjord (1988) likewise states, "My own clinical experience has also caused me to conclude that the role of external entities should be considered" (p. 135). Similarly, Canadian psychotherapist Adam Crabtree (1985), who is noted as a historian of mesmerism and dissociation, hints at such a possibility when describing his synthesis of the "occult" and "psychological" views of "multiple man." All three therapists have been known to report the use of exorcisms as a psychotherapeutic technique in some cases. It must also be acknowledged that all three clinicians are expressing a viewpoint that is controversial and exceptionally deviant when contrasted with the conventional views of mainstream medicine and psychiatry.

Multiple personality disorder is perhaps the hallmark of the group of mental disorders that were first given their own separate diagnostic category in 1980 in *DSM-III*, the dissociative disorders. The 1987 revision of the diagnostic manual (DSM-III-R) includes along with MPD psychogenic amnesia, depersonalization disorder, psychogenic fugue, and dissociative disorders not otherwise specified. "The essential feature of these disorders is a disturbance or alteration in the normally integrative functions of identity, memory, or consciousness" (American Psychiatric Association, 1987, p. 269). Certainly many of the case histories presented in this section fit within this category.

One interesting historical development has been reported by psychiatrist Philip Coons (1986), who was on the committee that was charged with the task to revise the section on dissociative disorders in the *DSM-III* for its next edition, which appeared in 1987. It seems that a century and a half after Esquirol proposed (unsuccessfully, as it turned out) that demonomania be considered a legitimate psychiatric diagnosis, in the 1980s many psychiatrists wanted to resurrect the idea as a proposed addition to the dissociative disorders in *DSM-III-R*. Prior to the publication of this revision, Coons (1986) reports:

> The work group to revise the psychiatric diagnostic manual, *DSM-III*, has proposed the addition of several other dissociative disorders. The first, trance/possession disorder, is marked by an altered state of consciousness and the belief that one has been taken over by a spirit or another person. This state occurs outside of a culturally sanctioned or religious context. Although such states have been reported throughout the world, until now they have not had a diagnostic category of their own. (pp. 412–413)

As it turned out, trance/possession disorder was not approved for the most recent version of what is reputed to be the most widely used diagnostic manual in the world, although some future edition may indeed include it. As the ancient Egyptians are famous for saying, there is indeed nothing new under the sun.

POSSESSION AS A CAUSE OF MENTAL DISORDER: C. G. JUNG

Of all the major 20th century theorists, only C. G. Jung openly and repeatedly cites possession as a cause of mental disorders. In fact, Jung is in agreement with several of the primitive concepts for the cause of disease cited in the introduction to this book and has incorporated them into his 20th century phenomenological psychology. Central to his use of this term is the phenomenology of mental life invoked by the complex theory and by one of its central processes, *dissociation*. An extensive treatment of the place of dissociation in Jung's complex theory and its relevance to multiple personality disorder has been given elsewhere (Noll, 1989), and therefore the reader is referred to that reference for further information.

Jung was fascinated by the "psychology of primitives" and taught university courses on that subject early in his career. He is also the only major figure in the psychology of personality to actually do his own anthropological fieldwork and did so on many occasions, most notably in the jungles of Africa and among the Pueblo Indians of the American Southwest. There are many elements of Jung's psychology that would be familiar to the shamans or witchdoctors or medicine men of nonliterate societies, as well as to the ancient or Medieval physicians of our own Western culture. Foremost among these concepts that would be familiar to the physicians of other times and other places is the notion that ego-alien forces can influence or, in some cases, totally supplant the volitional functioning of the ego and alter thoughts, feelings, and behaviors in remarkable ways.

As was briefly discussed in the previous section on lycanthropy, Jung considered the ego to be only one of a multitude of complexes. Each "feeling-toned complex" was a cluster of affects and images organized around a specific thematic core. Furthermore, each complex has an allotment of consciousness all of its own that is dissociated or split-off from the primary stream of consciousness which has the ego at its center as the primary organizational locus. These complexes arise from traumata as minor as a moral conflict (or perhaps breach of taboo in primitive terms) to as major as actual physical or sexual abuse or other forms of psychological duress. From the point of view of the ego, complexes are experienced as autonomous and ego-alien, and in some cases may even have identities all their own (as is especially found in multiple personality disorder). Jung therefore also calls complexes "splinter psyches."

Jung himself recognized how similar his complex theory was to primitive conceptions of mental health and disease: "To the uninitiated ear, my presentation of the complex theory may sound like a description of primitive demonology or of the psychology of taboos" (Jung, 1934/1948/1969, p.104). Indeed, Jung deliberately sought to ground his psychology in the anthropology of his day. Thus, an *anthropological* reading of Jung is crucial for understanding the broader implications of his psychology. For example, in his essay on "The Psychological Foundations of Belief in Spirits" (1920/1948/1969), Jung equates the primitive theory that some psychological or physical diseases are caused by the spirits of "certain persons, living or dead" (p. 304) with the powerful role played by the parental complexes in the symptoms of neurotic and psychotic disorders.

> As pathogenic conflicts usually go back to childhood and are connected with memories of the parents, we can understand why the primitive attaches special importance to the spirits of dead relatives. This accounts for the wide incidence of ancestor-worship, which is primarily a protection against the malice of the dead. Anyone who has had experience of nervous illnesses knows how great is the importance of parental influences on patients. Many patients feel persecuted by their parents long after they are dead. The psychological aftereffects of the parents are so powerful that many cultures developed a whole system of ancestor-worship to propitiate them. (Jung, 1920/1948/1969, p. 304)

In a footnote to this passage Jung relates a tale from his 1925–1926 expedition to Mount Elgon in East Africa about a native woman who became ill with what looked to Jung "like a septic abortion with high fever" (p. 394). Jung was unable to treat her adequately with the medical supplies on hand, and so her relatives called in a "medicine man" (*nganga*). According to Jung (p. 304), "When he arrived, the medicine-man walked round and round the hut in ever-widening circles, snuffing the air." The medicine-man then came to a halt on a path that led up to the nearby mountain, and told Jung and the woman's relatives that the spirits of the girl's parents—who both had died young—were now residing in a bamboo forest up on the mountain and would come down every night "to make their daughter ill so that she should die and keep them company." The medicine-man had them make a "ghost-trap" on the mountain path in the form of a little hut in which was placed a clay figure of the woman and some food, all of which was meant to trick the parental spirits into thinking they were with their daughter. The result? It worked. As Jung (p. 305) confesses, "To our boundless astonishment the girl recovered within two days. Was our diagnosis wrong? The puzzle remains unsolved."

Jung's references to possession are many, although they all express the same basic idea: "some content, an idea or part of the personality, obtains mastery of the individual for one reason or another" (Jung, 1940/1950/1968, p. 122). In one example Jung (1955/1970) lists "the symptoms of possession (such as compulsions, phobias, obsessions, automatisms, exaggerated affects, etc.)" (p. 180). In this regard he follows his teachers Janet and Freud, who, along with Breuer he credits for translating the medieval concept of possession into psychological language and for devising a therapeutic technique that resembled exorcism:

> The medieval theory of possession (toned down by Janet to "obsession") was thus taken over by Breuer and Freud in a more positive form, the evil spirit—to reverse the Faustian miracle—being transmogrified into a harmless "psychological formula." It is greatly to the credit of both investigators that they did not, like the rationalistic Janet, gloss over the significant analogy with possession, but rather, following the medieval theory, hunted up the factor causing the possession in order, as it were, to exorcise the evil spirit. Breuer was the first to discover that the pathogenic "ideas" were memories of certain events which he called "traumatic." . . . They realized that the symptom-producing "ideas" were rooted in an *affect*. This affect had the peculiarity of never really coming to the surface, so that it was never really conscious. The task of the therapist was therefore to "abreact" the "blocked" affect. (Jung, 1939/1966, p. 42)

Elsewhere Jung (1940/1950/1968) states that "possession can be formulated as the identity of the ego-personality with a complex" (p. 122). Also:

> When the unconscious contents are not "realized" they give rise to a negative activity and personification. . . . Psychic abnormalities then develop, states of possession ranging in ordinary moods and "ideas" to psychoses. All these states are characterized by one and the same fact that an unknown "something" has taken possession of a smaller or greater portion of the psyche and asserts its hateful and harmful existence undeterred by all our insight, reason, and energy, thereby proclaiming the power of the unconscious over the conscious mind. (Jung, 1928/1966, p. 370)

In 1945 Jung was asked to write an encyclopedia entry on the concept of demoniacal possession, of which only the first sentence was eventually published without attribution some years later. His submission is reproduced in full below and gives his clearest statement of this phenomenon:

> Demonism (synonymous with demonomania = possession) denotes a peculiar state of mind characterized by the fact that certain psychic contents, the so-called complexes, take over the control of the total personality in the place of the ego, at least temporarily, to such a degree that the free will of the ego is suspended. In certain of these states ego-consciousness is present, in others it is eclipsed. Demonism is a primordial psychic phenomenon and frequently occurs under primitive conditions. . . . The phenomenon of demonism is not always spontaneous, but can also be deliberately induced as a "trance," for instance in shamanism, spiritualism, etc. . . .
>
> Medically, demonism belongs partly to the sphere of the psychogenic neuroses, partly to that of schizophrenia. Demonism can also be epidemic. One of the most celebrated epidemics of the Middle Ages was the possession of the Ursulines of London, 1632. The epidemic form includes the induced collective psychoses of a religious or political nature,

such as those of the twentieth century. . . . (Jung, 1945/1976, p. 648)

A more current Jungian treatment of the Jungian concept of possession can be found in a volume by von Franz (1980), who was one of Jung's closest disciples and collaborators.

The case histories presented here, therefore, should be read with these overlapping interpretations in mind. There is no generally agreed-upon diagnostic criteria to definitely account for the phenomena discussed in the case histories below. Therefore, the readers of this volume are also asked to ponder the possibilities contemplated by Marescot and the physicians of Paris in the case of Marthe Brossier as they read the stories below: that is, whether these tales are due to "sicknesse, Counterfeiting, or Diabolicall possession" (cited in Walker, 1981, p. 37).

REFERENCES

Aldridge-Morris, R. (1989). *Multiple Personality: An Exercise in Deception.* Hillsdale, NJ: Lawrence Erlbaum.

Allison, R. (1980). *Minds in Many Pieces.* New York: Rawson, Wade.

American Psychiatric Association (1980). *Diagnostic and Statistical Manual of Mental Disorders, Third Edition.* Washington, D.C.: American Psychiatric Press.

American Psychiatric Association (1987). *Diagnostic and Statistical Manual of Mental Disorders, Third Edition, Revised.* Washington, D.C.: American Psychiatric Press.

Beahrs, J. O. (1982). *Unity and Multiplicity: Multilevel Consciousness of Self in Hypnosis, Psychiatric Disorder and Mental Health.* New York: Brunner/Mazel.

Bourguignon, E. (1973). *Religion, Altered States of Consciousness, and Social Change.* Columbus, OH: Ohio State University Press.

Bourguignon, E. (1976). *Possession.* San Francisco: Chandler & Sharp.

Brentano, F. (1874/1973). *Psychology From an Empirical Standpoint.* Oskar Kraus (Ed.). A. C. Rancurello, D. B. Terrell, & L. L. McAlister (Trans.). London: Routledge & Kegan Paul.

Coons, P. M. (1986, May). Dissociative disorders: Diagnosis and treatment. *Indiana Medicine*, pp. 410–415.

Crabtree, A. (1985). *Multiple Man: Explorations in Possession and Multiple Personality.* New York: Praeger.

Crapanzano, V., & Garrison, V. (1977). *Case Studies in Spirit Possession.* New York: John Wiley & Sons.

Ellenberger, H. (1970). *The Discovery of the Unconscious.* New York: Basic Books.

Esquirol, J. E. D. (1838/1845). *Mental Maladies. A Treatise on Insanity.* E. K. Hunt (Trans.). Philadelphia: Lea & Blanchard.

Goldstein, J. (1987). *Console and Classify: The French Psychiatric Profession in the Nineteenth Century.* Cambridge: Cambridge University Press.

Goodman, F. D. (Ed.) (1974). *Trance, Healing and Hallucination: Three Field Studies in Religious Existence.* New York: Wiley Interscience.

Goodman, F. D. (1981). *The Exorcism of Anneliese Michel.* New York: Doubleday.

Goodman, F. D. (1988). *How About Demons? Possession and Exorcism in the Modern World.* Bloomington: Indiana University Press.

Hilgard, E. R. (1986). *Divided Consciousness: Multiple Controls in Human Thought and Action.* 2nd ed. New York: John Wiley & Sons.

James, W. (1890). *The Principles of Psychology.* 2 vols. New York: Henry Holt.

Janet, P. (1889). *L'Automatisme Psychologique.* Paris: Felix Alcon.

Jung, C. G. (1920/1948/1969). The psychological foundations of a belief in spirits. In *The Structure and Dynamics of the Psyche. The Collected Works of C. G. Jung, Volume 8.* Princeton: Princeton University Press.

Jung, C. G. (1928/1966). The relations between the ego and the unconscious. In Jung, C. G., *Two Essays on Analytical Psychology. The Collected Works of C. G. Jung, Vol. 7.* Princeton: Princeton University Press.

Jung, C. G. (1934/1948/1969). A review of the complex theory. In *The Structure and Dynamics of the Psyche. The Collected Works of C. G. Jung, Volume 8.* Princeton: Princeton University Press.

Jung, C. G. (1939/1966). In memory of Sigmund Freud. In Jung, C. G., *The Spirit in Man, Art, and Literature. The Collected Works of C. G. Jung, Vol. 15.* Princeton: Princeton University Press.

Jung, C. G. (1940/1950/1968). Concerning rebirth. In Jung, C. G., *The Archetypes of the Collected Unconscious. The Collected Works of C. G. Jung, Vol. 9, I.* Princeton: Princeton University Press.

Jung, C. G. (1945/1976). The definition of demonism. In Jung, C. G., *The Symbolic Life: Miscellaneous Writings. The Collected Works of C. G. Jung, Vol. 18.* Princeton: Princeton University Press.

Jung, C. G. (1970). *Mysterium Conjunctionis. The Collected Works of C. G. Jung, Vol. 14.* Princeton: Princeton University Press.

Kelly, H. A. (1968). *The Devil, Demonology and Witchcraft: The Development of Christian Beliefs in Evil Spirits.* Garden City, NY: Doubleday.

Kemp, S. (1990). *Medieval Psychology.* Westport, CT: Greenwood.

Kemp, S., & Williams, K. (1987). Demonic possession and mental disorder in medieval and early modern Europe. *Psychological Medicine, 17,* 21–29.

Kenny, M. G. (1986). *The Passion of Ansel Bourne: Multiple Personality in American Culture.* Washington, D.C.: Smithsonian Institution Press.

Lewis, I. M. (1971). *Ecstatic Religion: An Anthropological Study of Spirit Possession and Shamanism.* Middlesex, England: Penguin.

Lewis, I. M. (1986). *Religion in Context: Cults and Charisma.* Cambridge: Cambridge University Press.

Myers, F. W. H. (1903). *Human Personality and Its Survival of Bodily Death.* 2 vols. London: Longman, Greens, & Co.

Naegeli-Osjord, H. (1988). *Possession and Exorcism.* Oregon, WI: New Frontiers Center.

Noll, R. (1989). Multiple personality, dissociation, and C. G. Jung's complex theory. *Journal of Analytical Psychology, 34*, 353–370.

Oesterreich, T. K. (1935). *Obsession and Possession by Spirits both Good and Evil.* D. Ibberson (trans.). Chicago: The de Laurence Company.

Pinel, P. (1801/1806). *A Treatise on Insanity.* D. D. David (trans.). Sheffield, England.

Prince, R. (Ed.) (1968). *Trance and Possession States.* Montreal: R. M. Bucke Memorial Society.

Putnam, F. W. (1989). *Diagnosis and Treatment of Multiple Personality Disorder.* New York: Guilford.

Quen, J. M. (Ed.) (1986). *Split Minds, Split Brains: Historical and Current Perspectives.* New York: New York University Press.

Rosen, G. (1968). *Madness in Society: Chapters in the Historical Sociology of Mental Illness.* Chicago: University of Chicago Press.

Ross, C.A. (1989). *Multiple Personality Disorder: Diagnosis, Clinical Features, and Treatment.* New York: John Wiley & Sons.

Spanos, N. P., & Gottlieb, J. (1979). Demonic possession, mesmerism, and hysteria: A social psychological perspective and their historical interrelations. *Journal of Abnormal Psychology, 88*, 527–546.

Taylor, E. (1982). *William James on Exceptional Mental States: The 1896 Lowell Lectures.* New York: Scribner's.

Temkin, O. (1945). *The Falling Sickness. A History of Epilepsy from the Greeks to the Beginnings of Modern Neurology.* Baltimore:Johns Hopkins University Press.

von Franz, M. L. (1980). *Projection and Re-Collection in Jungian Psychology: Reflections of the Soul.* La Salle, IL: Open Court.

Walker, D. P. (1981). *Unclean Spirits: Possession and Exorcism in France and England in the Late Sixteenth and Early Seventeenth Centuries.* Philadelphia: University of Pennsylvania Press.

Zilboorg, G. (1941). *A History of Medical Psychology.* New York: Norton.

11

Demonomania

J. E. D. ESQUIROL

Origin, history and signification of term.—Origin of religious melancholy.—Stellar and lunar influence.—Influence of the doctrine of the Platonists on mental alienation.—Origin of conjurations, sorcery, magic, witchcraft and astrology.—Influence of Christianity on the form and treatment of insanity.—The effect of the reformation of Luther and Calvin.—Mode of dissipating the errors which led to this form of insanity.—Analysis of symptoms of this malady, compared with those that attend other forms of melancholy.—Case.—Post-mortem examination.—Cases.—Sometimes epidemic.—Examples.—Demoniacal possession rarely occurs before puberty.—Women more subject to this disease than men.—Causes, physical and moral.—Its access generally sudden.—Demonomaniacs usually emaciated, etc.—Exhale a strong odor.—Ecstasies common, and modified by various circumstances.—Demonomaniacs suffer from hallucinations and illusions.—Case.—Tenacious of their delusions.—Examples.—Tests of demoniacal possession.—Death often hailed with joy by the possessed.—Convulsions not uncommon.—Important conclusions.—Suicide much to be feared in this form of insanity.—Of all insane persons, lypemaniacs are the most cruel.—Treatment.—Medical.—

Reprinted from *Mental Maladies. A Treatise on Insanity.* Translated from the French, with additions, by E. K. Hunt, M.D. Philadelphia: Lea and Blanchard, 1845.

Moral.—Zoanthropy.—Lycanthropy.—Fatalists, or believers in destiny.—Several strange views referred to.—Examples, with a post-mortem examination.

The word demon among the ancients, was not understood in a bad sense. It signified the Divinity, a tutelary Genius, a guardian Spirit; δαίμονιθν, is derived from δαίμων, sapiens, sciens. Plato assigned this name to that Spirit with whom the Supreme Being intrusted the government of the world. The Jews, after the Chaldeans, attributed almost all diseases to the agency of spirits or demons. Saul is troubled by an evil spirit; Job is the sport of a demon. The dysentery which smote Joram, was referred to the same cause. Nebuchadonosor is seized with lycanthropy by the command of God. Is it astonishing that hysteria, epilepsy and melancholy are called *sacred*? The Greeks also, charged the spirits with being the cause of the major part of their diseases. Herodotus affirms, that Cleomenes did not become furious in consequence of the presence of demons, but because he was intoxicated with the Scythians. Aristophanes denominates the most intense degree of fury, not μανία, but χαχοδαίμονία. By preserving the primitive signification of this word, we should have given the name of demonomania to religious melancholy. The first variety of this form of insanity would have designated that class of insane, who believe that they are God, who imagine that they have conversations and intimate communications with the Holy Spirit, angels and saints, and who pretend to be inspired, and to have received a commission from heaven to convert men. This species would have been denominated *theomania*; while the second would have been called *cacodemonomania*, and would have embraced all those unfortunate beings who fancied that they were possessed by the devil, and in his power; who were convinced that they had been present at the imaginary assemblies of evil spirits, or who feared damnation, and the misery of eternal fire. This classification would present, in a single variety, all those forms of delirium which have reference to religious beliefs. It would place in opposition all the varieties of religious melancholy; while the religious, gay and bold forms of delirium, attended with pride and exaltation of the faculties, would be, so to speak, placed in comparison with the sad and timid forms, attended by despondency and terror. But the word *demonomania* is appropriated; and the public would charge me with neologism, were I to restore it to its etymological signification.

Man, dependent by his organization upon external influences, and passing alternately from well-being to sorrow, from pain to pleasure, and from fear to hope, was naturally led to reflect upon the nature and relations of good and evil. He soon admitted the existence of a good being, and a malevolent spirit, which presided over his good or ill fortune. A step more only, and a system of theology was formed. Religion was now, gentle and full of consolation; now, she assumed a severe and threatening tone. But sorrow having pervaded almost the entire existence of man, and pain being more extensively prevalent in the world, ideas of a depressing character predominated. From sadness, to fear and terror, there was but a step. These sentiments inspired in the earliest period of the world, a sort of religious melancholy, depending upon those fearful terrors that had their origin with the birth of the world. Religious melancholy was, therefore, of all forms of mental alienation, the most general and extended. The sacred books of every people present examples of it. When man, abandoning the worship of the true God, fell into idolatry, the first objects of his adoration were the stars. (Newton, chronol.) These most strongly impressed his senses, and exercised over him the most active and long-continued influence. Religious melancholy was regarded as dependent upon the course of the stars, and its periodicity strengthened this belief. The insane were called maniacs, a word derived from μηνη, *luna, lune*, from which the Greeks made *maniacs*, moon-struck, and the Latins *lunatics*; an appellation which is still maintained in England, and also in France, in the language of common life. When the doctrine of spirits, taught by the Platonists, at length complicates their theological notions, nervous maladies, and particularly mental alienation, being sacred diseases, were attributed to the agency of spirits and demons. Among the insane, some were gay, bold and rash, regarding themselves as inspired. They believed themselves fortunate, and the friends of the gods; and presented themselves, or were presented to the people, as those sent from heaven. They also uttered oracles on their own, and on account of the priests. Others, on the contrary, sad, timid, pusillanimous, fearful, and pursued by imaginary terrors, pronounced themselves condemned forever. They were treated as objects of celestial wrath, and regarded themselves as devoted to the powers of hell. Meleager, Œdipus and Orestes, and many other illustrious subjects of divine wrath, were pursued by furies. These were true lypemaniacs.

Disquietude, fear or fright, modified or changed the nature of all.

They deemed it necessary to deliver themselves from some extraordinary evil, or to turn aside the vengeance of the gods. They desired also to read in the future, what they were to fear or to hope for. They evoked the souls of the dead, after having consulted the oracles and stars. The followers of Orpheus gave birth to the science of conjurations, sorcery, and many other mysterious practices. Magic and witchcraft formed a part of their religious worship. Sovereigns, legislators and philosophers, were initiated into the mysteries; some, to extend the sphere of their knowledge, and others, from motives as shameful as criminal. Astrology, magic and witchcraft, all children of fear, so enchained the imagination of men, that we need not be astonished, says Pliny, that their influence lasts so long, and has extended to all ages, regions and people. Christianity, by recalling religious views to the unity of God, by causing oracles to cease, and by enlightening men, rendered sacred the opinions of Plato and Socrates, respecting the existence of demons, and wrought a great revolution in the sentiments of men. They exaggerated the power of spirits over matter, and the fear of yielding to the instigations of the devil, created dread. They believed that from the commencement of this life, they were in the power of demons, and the number of demonomaniacs multiplied. This, the institution of exorcisms in the primitive church establishes. They had recourse to ceremonies and prayers to deliver the possessed, but did not burn them. They established, in several cities, solemn feasts for the cure of the possessed. They were accustomed to assemble in a church all the insane of a country, whither they came from the most remote regions. The concourse of people, assembled from every quarter, the presence of the bishop, the pomp and solemn display, the confidence which took possession of the sick, and every thing that could control their imagination, contributed to the cure of some of these unfortunate beings. They proclaim it a miracle, and this persuasion prepared new cures for succeeding years. These solemnities, which, in some cities of France were still celebrated so late as the middle of the last century, must not be confounded with what they called the *feast of mad-people*, a strange saturnal, which took place in certain chapters, during the fourteenth and fifteenth centuries.

When the impetuous Luther, on pretext of removing abuses, attempted to revolutionize the church in order to avenge his quarrels, religious discussions became the subject of all conversations, of all sermons, and even of all political reports. The diverse parties, reciprocally menaced each other with eternal damnation. Fanaticism was aroused, and religious melancholy added to all those ills that innovations had provoked. Calvin augmented them still more. We see none but the excommunicated, the condemned and wizards. The public were alarmed, created tribunals, the devil was summoned to appear, the possessed were brought to judgment. They erected scaffolds, and kindled funeral piles. Demonomaniacs, under the name of sorcerers and possessed, victims in a double sense of the prevailing errors, were burnt, after having been put to the torture in order to induce them to renounce their pretended *compact* with the devil. In these unhappy times, such was the mania for attributing every thing to the agency of the devil, that Pierre de L'Ancre, not being able to comprehend how a rock, situated near a village of Asia, called *Arpasa*, of which Pliny speaks, and which, like the rock of Cydobre among the Albigenses, moves when one touches it with the end of the finger, while the most powerful efforts failed in producing this result, attributes this phenomenon to the power of a demon. G. E. Stahl* relates cases of grave maladies, which were regarded as the work of the devil.

Were this the place for it, I could prove that the insane had been employed to utter oracles, and that the priests knew how to inspire themselves with a holy delirium. I shall show farther on, that demoniacal possession is a true monomania. Demons became mute from the time that Christianity shed its benign influences abroad over the world†. They ceased to plague men, so soon as men ceased to fear. They no sooner ceased to burn sorcerers and magicians, than the imagination became composed, and no longer gave birth to either of them. Many now fear the police, as they would formerly have done the stars and demons. This fear is so much the more intense and fatal, as the police acquires more influence in times of trouble and civil dissensions; and we shall no longer be surprised, if in hospitals for the insane, demonomaniacs are replaced by a class which fears the police, prison and punishment. It is ever the weakness of the human mind, pusillanimity, disquietude and fear, which acts upon these unfortunate beings, producing such results as were formerly regarded as demoniacal possession. That man is now in a mad-house, because he fears the police, who would formerly have been burnt because he feared the devil.

---

*Collegium causale sic dictim minus. Swidnitü, 1734, in 4to.
†Fontenelle, History of Oracles, in 12mo.

Physicians, and some men of superior wisdom, have, in all times, combatted the prejudices which caused the true sources of nervous maladies and mental alienation to be overlooked. Hippocrates or his disciples, in the treatise "*On the Sacred Disease*," assures us, that there can be no maladies caused by the gods. Areteus expresses the same sentiment. *De causis morb. diut*, lib. I. The report of Marescot, Riolan and Duret, respecting the possession of Martha Brossier, is a model of sound reason and wisdom. They reduce their opinion to these memorable terms: *nihil a demone; multa ficta, a morbo pauca.* "Nothing from the devil; many things feigned: few things from disease." Cardan, Corneille Looz, Joseph Duchêne, Bekker, Pigray, Bayle, Naude and Mead, defended these unfortunate beings against both the prejudiced and the Del-Rios, Bodins, Pierre de l'Ancres, etc. Malebranche, whose opinion should not be suspected, speaks with a noble boldness.* Parliaments, under the presidency of Seguier, annulled many decrees, which condemned to the flames both sorcerers and the possessed. All have read that beautiful passage of Aguesseau, where this celebrated magistrate says to parliament, that in order to cause sorcery to cease, all that is necessary is, no longer to speak of sorcerers, and to attribute no kind of importance to the matter, but to commit, without noise, to the physicians, the wizards, who were "more sinned against, than sinning." Both sorcerers and the possessed were, in fact, often the victims of impostors, who made traffic of the ignorance and superstition of their fellow creatures. They were imbeciles, melancholics and hysterical persons, who were believed to be possessed, because they had been threatened with demons and wizards; and judges doomed these unhappy beings to the flames. A jurisprudence existed, having reference to sorcery and magic, as laws were enacted against robbery and murder. The people, seeing both Church and prince believe in the reality of these extravagances, remained invincibly persuaded. The more they pursued sorcerers and the possessed, and the more ceremony attended their punishment, the more was the number of these persons augmented, by exciting the imagination, and occupying it with chimerical fears. A better education and the progress of knowledge, have gradually dissipated these fatal errors, more successfully than funeral piles, or legal code and digest.

Though demonomania may be unusual at this day, it will not be unin-

*Researches Concerning Truth; Paris, 1762, 4 vol. in 12mo.

teresting to point out and determine its characters. If the possessed no longer exist, there are still some monomaniacs who consider themselves in the power of the devil. I have collected certain facts respecting demonomania, and have compared them with what demonographers have related. Their resemblance has satisfied me that the symptoms that I observed are the same, with the signs of possession pointed out by authors, or contained in the accounts of the trials of sorcerers and those possessed. After having given a brief history of demonomania, we will pass on to an analysis and comparison of the symptoms of this malady, with those that attend other forms of melancholy.

A. D., a servant woman forty-six years of age, was of medium size, had chestnut colored hair, small hazel eyes, a dark complexion, and an ordinary degree of fullness of habit. Endowed with great susceptibility, she has much self-esteem, and was religiously educated. Fourteen years of age. First menstruation, and since that period the menses have been scanty and irregular. Thirty years. She becomes attached to a young man, whom they will not permit to marry her. She becomes sad and melancholic, believing herself abandoned by every body. The menses cease, not to appear again. She engages with extreme ardor in devotional exercises, makes a vow of chastity, and devotes herself to Jesus Christ. Sometime after this, she fails in her promises, and remorse seizes upon her. She regards herself as condemned, given over to the evil one, and suffers the torments of hell. Six years she passes in this state of delirium and torments; after which, exercise, dissipation and the influence of time, restore her to reason and her ordinary occupations. Forty years of age. Forsaken by a new lover, D. renews her vows of chastity, and passes her time in prayer. One day, while on her knees reading the imitation of Jesus Christ, a young man enters her chamber, says that he is Jesus Christ, that he has come to console her, and that if she will but trust in him, she will have no longer occasion to fear the devil. She yields. For the second time she considers herself in the power of the devil, and experiences all the torments of hell and despair. Sent to the Salpêtrière, she spends most of her time in bed, groaning night and day, eating little, continually complaining, and relating her misfortunes to all. Forty-six years of age, March 16th, 1813. This woman is transferred to the infirmary for the insane. Her emaciation is extreme, skin earthy, face pale and convulsive, the eyes dull and fixed; the breath fetid, the tongue dry, rough, and interspersed with whitish points. She refuses nourishment, although she says that she is tormented by hunger and thirst. There is insomnia, together with a small and feeble pulse, head heavy, with a burning sensation internally, and a feeling as if bound with a cord externally. There is a painful constriction of the throat, and she is constantly rolling up the skin of her neck with her fingers, and crowding it behind the sternum; assuring us that the devil draws it, and that he strangles and prevents her from swallowing any thing. There is considerable tension of the muscles of the abdomen, attended by constipation; and upon the back of the right hand and left foot, are scrofulous tumors. The devil has extended a cord from the sternum to the pubes, which prevents the patient from standing up. He is in her body, burning and pinching it. He also gnaws her heart, and rends her entrails. She is surrounded by flames, and in the midst of the fires of hell, though we see them not. No one may credit it, but her ills are unprecedented, frightful, eternal. She is damned. Heaven can have no compassion upon her.

April, 1813, diminution of the vital forces. The patient sees no one who approaches her. Day appears to her a light, in the midst of which wander spectres and demons, which reproach her for her conduct, threaten and maltreat her. She refuses all consolation, and becomes irritated if we persist in offering it. The assistance of the ministers of religion is useless, and the aid of medicine rejected. This malady being never seen, men can do nothing; a supernatural power is necessary. She curses the devil, who burns and tortures her, and God, who has cast her into hell. May 1813; marasmus, abdominal members retracted upon the abdomen; decline of the vital forces, though the patient often says that she can never die. May 25th; tongue brown, burning heat, difficult respiration, thirst, pulse small and contracted. May 30th: feet swollen, chills at irregular intervals, though she has at the same time sensations of heat. Mournful groans. June 6th. A serious diarrhœa, feet swollen at times, the cheeks very much flushed, the tongue black, the skin earthy, pulse very small and frequent. June 15th: prostration, eschar over the coccyx, delirium the same. June 21st: aphonia, respiration frequent, pulse scarcely perceptible; the same groans, the same delirium, and conviction that she should not die. June 22nd. Death took place at seven o'clock in the evening; for two days previous to this event, she could execute no movement, and swallowed nothing.

June 24th. Post-mortem examination: marasmus, feet edematous, lower extremities retracted, eschars on the coccyx and sacrum. Cranium thickened anteriorly, diploe injected. Falciform fold of the duramater reticulated, and torn anteriorly. Serum at the base of the cranium. Some points of ossification in the Pineal gland. Cerebrum and cerebellum softened, grey substance pale. Serum abundant in the two lateral and third ventricles; plexus chorrides discolored, having many small, serous cysts. Very extended adhesions of the posterior portions of the two ventricles. Lungs tuberculous, and adherent throughout their whole extent to the pleuræ. A small quantity of serum in the pericardium, to which the right auricle and point of the heart adhere. Epiploon atrophied, and interspersed with small black points, as was also the peritoneum throughout its whole extent. All the abdominal viscera, adhering closely together, form but a single mass of a brownish aspect; mesenteric glands very much developed, and some of them, as large as hazel nuts, are converted into adipocere. The gall-bladder contains little bile, the spleen is reduced to the consistence of pap and the color of lees of wine; the mucous membrane of the intestines is ulcerated in several points, and that of the urinary bladder reddish. The forehead is retreating, and very narrow from temple to temple. The excessive flattening of the coronal region, gives to this profile one of the characters which have been pointed out as proper to idiocy.

M., now forty-nine years of age, living in the country, and a wool-spinner by occupation, had often heard accounts of sorcerers. At fifteen years of age, the menses appear spontaneously. Thirty-seven. When on the point of marriage, she learns that her pretended lover is deceiving her. She will no longer listen to him, and a year after marries another person. He whom she has forsaken, threatens her with vengeance, and dooms her to the dwelling place of devils. A man in the village where she resides, who passes for a sorcerer, gives his body, without the least doubt on her part, to the devil. At forty years of age the menses cease. At this period her ideas become deranged, but in a manner imperceptible to strangers, and she suffers from cephalalgia. Forty-two years. Returning from a long excursion, she is fatigued, and lies down upon the earth to refresh herself. Shortly after, she experiences in her head a motion and noise like that of a spinning wheel. She is frightened, but nevertheless resumes her course, and on the way, is raised from the earth, to the height of more than seven feet. Having reached her place of residence, she can neither eat nor drink. She calls to mind the threat that had been made with reference to her, four years previously, and no longer doubts that she is bewitched. Many remedies are administered, and she makes prayers, performs devotions of nine days' duration, and also pilgrimages. She wears a stole, which had been presented her by a priest. But all in vain. The devil and his torments no longer leave her, and three years afterwards, she is brought to the Salpêtrière.

At the time of her arrival at the hospital she is extremely emaciated, her skin is sun-burnt, earthy, and hot; the pulse is feeble and small, the head is bowed down, the face bloated, and the forehead wrinkled. The eye-brows, at times mingling with the folds of the forehead, are lost in the hair: the abdomen is hard and voluminous, and the patient has her hand constantly upon it. She assures us that she has, in her uterus, an evil spirit, in the form of a serpent, which leaves her neither day nor night, although her organs of generation are not like those of other women. She complains of a great degree of constriction about the throat, and experiences a necessity to walk about, and suffers much more acutely if prevented from doing so. She walks slowly, speaking in a low tone of her condition, which she deplores. She conceals herself when she eats and drinks, as well as when called to evacuate the bladder and bowels, in order to better persuade us that she is not a body, but merely a spectre and imaginary being.

"The devil has taken from me my body, and I have no longer a human shape. There is nothing so dreadful as to appear to live and yet not to be of this world. I burn, sulphur exhales with my breath. I neither eat or drink, because the devil has no need either of food or drink. I feel nothing, and should I be placed in a terrestrial fire, I should not burn. I shall live millions of years; that which is upon the earth not being able to die. Were it not so, despair would have caused me, long since, to terminate my existence."

Nothing undeceives her, and she is abusive in her language to those who seem to doubt the truth of what she affirms. Those who contradict her, she calls sorcerers and demons. If they insist upon the correctness of their opinion respecting her, she becomes irritated, her eyes project, and are red and haggard. Look then, she says, at this beautiful figure; is it that of a woman or a devil? She strikes herself violently with her fist upon her chest. She pretends also, to be insensible, and to prove it, pinches her skin with all her might, and strikes her chest with a wooden shoe. I have myself pinched her, pricked her often with a pin, and transfixed the skin of her arm, without her testifying the least suffering. Still she manifested pain when not forewarned. This woman is tranquil, is not mischievous, and speaks rationally upon every other subject, when we can divert her thoughts. On pretext of delivering her out of the power of the devil, and unbewitching her, she was thrice magnetized, but without my being able to witness any magnetic effect.

H., fifty-one years of age, and a peddler by occupation, menstruated only after the age of twenty-four years. She is subject to a headache and colic pains, and is the mother of three children. At the age of thirty-six years, and during her last pregnancy, she was accustomed to read the Apocalypse, and books which treated of ghosts and wizards. She was often frightened by these readings. Her last confinement was laborious, and she afterwards had several fainting turns. From time to time, she seemed to see flames. When thirty-seven years old, she borrows some money to oblige a relative. The creditor harasses and threatens her. Distressed by this debt, and while walking in the garden connected with her residence, the devil appears to her, proposes to her to sign a paper with blood drawn from the little finger of her left hand, and promises her the sum of money she owes. After a long debate, she writes out her renunciation of God, and her voluntary sacrifice to the devil. No sooner has she committed this act, than the earth trembles beneath her feet and around her. Her house also, is encompassed by a whirlwind, which shakes and injures its roof. At this instant, the evil spirit disappears, carrying away with him her real body, leaving only a phantom. All her neighbors were terrified witnesses of these phenomena. Her real body being with the devil, its image is tempted to throw itself into the water, and to strangle itself. The devil incites her to divers crimes. Feeling that she was devoured by the fires of hell, she threw herself into a pond, and suffers more since than before. She has no blood, and is absolutely insensible. I pierced through the skin of her arm with a pin, but she appeared to experience no pain in consequence of it. I shall remain upon the earth, she says, until wise men have discovered a means of obliging the devil to bring back to the earth my natural body. All that I say was taught me by the body which no longer exists, but which, before my misfortune, was upon the earth.

This woman is very much emaciated, her skin very brown and sunburnt. Grief and despair are depicted upon her countenance, which is wrinkled and contracted. She walks about quietly, knitting, and avoids her companions. She does not regard herself as sick, but groans about her miserable condition, which nothing can change. She is tranquil, supports opposition, and has a great desire to be relieved of her infirmity. Cherishing this hope, she has four times consented to be magnetized, without however, deriving the least possible effect from the operation. With the expectation that her portrait would be carried to the archbishop, she places herself in a very proper attitude to have it taken. Such was the condition of this unfortunate woman for twelve years. During eleven of them, she performed laborious services, fulfilling her duties very satisfactorily. For one year only, did age and wretchedness compel her to enter the Salpêtrière.

L. is fifty seven years of age, a laundress, and has been very devout from infancy. Menstruation commences at the age of fifteen years. At the age of seventeen she is married, and becomes the mother of fifteen children. When forty-six years of age, she loses her husband and one of her children, which expires in her arms; since which period, there have been anomalies with respect to menstruation. Near this time, she indulges in religious scruples; accuses herself of having partaken of the sacrament unworthily; takes an exaggerated view of religious exercises; neglects her occupations; and passes her time in the church. There is insomnia. She groans and stands in fear of hell. Fifty-two years of age. Cessation of the menses. Her fears are converted into religious terror, and she believes herself to be in the power of the devil. Fifty-four years of age; fever and delirium. She throws herself from the window, and is sent to the Hôtel-Dieu, from whence, after five months, she is transferred to the Salpêtrière. Extreme emaciation, skin sun-burnt, earthy, and complexion sallow. Expression of countenance restless. The whole body is in a sort of vacillation and continual balancing. She is constantly walking about, seeking to do mischief; to strike, to kill.

"For a million of years I have been the wife of the devil. I know that I am with him; for he lodges with me, and ceases not to say to me, that he is the father of my children. I suffer from uterine pains. My body is a sac, made of the skin of the devil, and is full of toads, serpents, and other unclean beasts, which spring from devils. I have no occasion to eat (though she eats largely). All that is given me is poison. I should long since have been dead, were I not the devil. For more than twenty years I have had no alvine evacuation. I have committed every kind of crime; have slain and robbed. The devil is continually telling me to slay, and even to strangle my children. In one minute, I commit more crimes than all rogues have committed in a hundred years. Hence I am not sorry to wear a strait waistcoat; for without this precaution, I should be dangerous. In giving myself away to the devil, I have been constrained to devote my children to him. But in return, I have required the devil to bring low, him that sits on high; to slay God, and the Virgin. When I was accustomed to receive the sacrament, I treated with contempt the good God of the Church. I no longer believe in him; it is no longer necessary for me to do so. It is no longer necessary to make confession, the devil forbids."

L. remains aside, avoids her companions, fears lest she shall do them harm, talks to herself, sees the devil on every side, and often disputes with him. This unhappy being presents an example of demonomania, complicated with dementia and fury. The strangest illusions and hallucinations maintain her delirium, and provoke acts of the blindest fury.

S., forty-eight years of age, is devoured by two demons who have taken up their abode in her haunches, and come forth through her ears. Devils have made several marks upon her person, and her heart is daily displaced. She shall never die, though the devil may tell her to go and drown herself. She has seen the two devils by which she is possessed. They are cats; one of which is yellow and white, and the other black. She puts tobacco, wine, and particularly grease, upon her head and in her ears, to exorcise the devil. She walks constantly with naked feet in fair and rainy weather, and while walking, picks up whatever comes in her way. She mislays her clothing, eats largely, and the dejections are involuntary. She sleeps not, is filthy, emaciated, and her skin very much sun-burnt. There is no coherence, even in the system of ideas that constantly occupy her mind. She articulates sounds with the greatest difficulty. This is a striking case of demonomania, which has degenerated into dementia, complicated with paralysis.

I may be censured for having multiplied cases. However, even in their abridgment, they have appeared to me to offer the more interest, as the first three furnish us an example of simple demonomania, and the two latter, that of this malady complicated with dementia; the one attended with fury, the other with paralysis. Besides, the whole five present features which characterize demoniacal possession. I pass to the analysis and appreciation of the symptoms of this malady, compared with the signs of possession, pointed out by writers on demonology. Demonomania is sometimes epidemic. Like all nervous maladies, it propagates itself by a kind of moral contagion, and by the power of imitation. The *mal des andous*, which afflicted Holland, Belgium and Germany, in the fourteenth century, was a kind of demonomania. In 1552 or 54, there was at Rome an epidemic of the possessed, which affected eighty-four persons. A franciscan monk exorcised them in vain. The devils accused the Jews. The major part of those possessed were Jewish women who had been baptized. About the same period, in the monastery of Kerndrop in Germany, all the nuns were possessed. The devils designated the cook of the convent, who confessed that she was a sorceress, and was burnt, together with her mother. The neighboring villages were also infected. The example of the possessed at Loudun, indicated most clearly, the power of the imagination and imitation. This epidemic having pervaded certain neighboring cities, threatened the Cevennes and all Upper Languedoc; when the prudent policy of a bishop checked the progress of the evil, by divesting it of whatever pertained to the marvelous, with which the imagination had furnished it. The convulsionists of St. Medard, deservedly figure among the victims of moral contagion. This happily, is the last scene of the kind that has afflicted our country.

We have elsewhere seen, that delirium ordinarily takes the character of the ideas prevailing at the epoch when the insanity bursts forth. So demonomania is most frequent when religious ideas occupy the mind, and are the subject of all discussions, whether public or private, civil or political. The history of Christianity, the irruption of the religion of Mahomet, and the establishment of Lutheranism and Calvinism prove this. In our day, the delirium of many insane persons runs upon politics. Mental alienation is strikingly hereditary. Why should not demonomania be so also? Should we be surprised, if writers on demonology tell us, that from generation to generation, the members of the same family were devoted to the devil, or were sorcerers?

Very rarely were they accustomed to see cases of demoniacal possession, previous to the age of puberty. Although a father and mother might have devoted their children to the devil, before or soon after their birth, they were initiated or admitted to the assembly of witches only after the age of puberty. Before this period of life, there was neither mania nor melancholy. The age most favorable for possession is from forty to fifty years. Old persons are little exposed to it. Thus, all authors observe that old men are no better adapted to utter oracles than for sorcery. An enfeebled imagination no longer lends itself to these miserable illusions. The appellation of *old sorceress*, confirms this result of general observation. One of the influences of this *old sorceress* is shown by a dry, emaciated, wrinkled and decrepit exterior, in the case of demonomaniacs who, in consequence of the moral tortures which they experience, and the physical evils and privations they endure, grow old, long before the usual decay of nature. Women are more subject to this disease than men. Pliny assures us, that women are to be preferred to men, in magic. Quintilian is of the same opinion. Saul goes to consult witches. Those are witches whom the Jewish records recommend us to guard against. They were priestesses, pythonissæ and sybils, who uttered oracles. Bodin maintains that at the most, we find but one sorcerer to fifty sorceresses. Paul Zacchias establishes a still greater difference. Woman is more decidedly nervous; she is more dependent upon her imagination, more submissive to the effects of fear and fright, more accessible to religious notions, more given to the marvelous, more subject to melancholy than man. Having reached the critical period, forsaken by the world, and passing from ennui to sadness, woman sinks into lypemania, often into its religious form. If hysteria be blended with it, the conflict of the senses with the religious principles, plunges her into demonomania, when mental weakness, ignorance and prejudices have, so to speak, fashioned the mind in advance, for a similar disease.

The melancholic temperament, as that most favorable for the production of lypemania, is that of the greater part of demonomaniacs. A nervous habit, an imagination easily excited, and a pusillanimous disposition, essentially predispose to this disease. It would be difficult to point out the conditions of life most favorable to the development of lypemania. It embraces among its victims, sovereigns, legislators, philosophers, the learned; but more particularly the ignorant; men, whose infancy has been spent in listening to the histories of wizards, demons, ghosts, and all those influences that are calculated to keep the mind restless, tormented, and disposed to the strangest impressions of alarm and fear. (Mallebranche). A bad education, religious fanaticism, an ascetic life, false and exaggerated notions of divine justice, damnation and hell, are also causes, more or less remote, of this disease; just as the perusal of romances disposes to erotic melancholy, and the reading of mystical books, or those relating to sorcery, to demonomania. For a long period, demonomania has been scarcely observed, and attacks only the feeble-minded and credulous. Since the reign of Henry III, Œrodius remarks that sorcery has been the portion only of the ignorant and peasantry. Among more than twenty thousand insane persons who have passed under my observation, I have scarcely seen one among a thousand, stricken with this fatal disease. They are, almost invariably, persons belonging to the lowest class of society; rarely men occupying rank in the world by their birth, education and fortune. There are besides, certain worthless knaves, who abuse the simplicity and ignorance of the inhabitants of the country, by causing them to believe that they possess a diabolical power; that they can destroy the virile power; make children sick; and throw a spell over the flocks. Certain phenomena imperfectly observed, fortify the belief of these timid, simple and credulous people, and sorcery still maintains certain obscure and contemptible relics of its ancient power. We still find in Germany, certain traces of this leprosy of the human mind, which, with this exception, is banished into the extreme north of Europe; and into the country of the Malaquais, Siamese, Indians, and other people enveloped in the thick darkness of ignorance.

The individual and proximate causes of demonomania, are the same with those of lypemania; but this variety recognizes causes which may be regarded as specific. They are either physical or moral. A feeble mind, a vicious education, the reading of works on sorcery, magic, etc.; false religious notions and prejudices, predispose to demonomania. An intense moral commotion, a fright, an unusual or threatening proposal or look, an exciting sermon, the force of imitation, suffice to produce an attack. Widowhood, the critical period, frictions upon the body, suppositories prepared from certain substances, drinks composed of enervating and narcotic substances; such are the physical causes of this malady. Gassendi tells us, that a provincial shepherd was accustomed to provide himself with a suppository of *Stramonium* when he retired at night, and on waking would relate all that he had seen at the witch-meeting. Certain sorcerers in order to gain access to these assemblages, were accustomed to anoint their bodies with fat, which had been prepared with irritating, or narcotic substances. These applications produce their effects in two ways: 1st, upon the imagination: by exciting and fixing it upon events, promised and desired; 2d, by irritating the brain, they provoked dreams, which were almost always predicated upon the ideas, desires or fears of the sleeper. This mode of enchantment is very ancient, since the Greeks denominated sorcerers and magicians φαϱϱαχίδεζ. They also gave them this name perhaps because the use of plants was connected with their enchantments.

Demoniacal possession has often been caused by the look merely, of a sorcerer. The influence of an amorous look upon a young person, the effects of a choleric or threatening expression upon a timid or prejudiced mind; will they not account for the consequences of enchantment by the *look!* without the necessity of having recourse to a supernatural and diabolical power? The attack of demonomania bursts forth, in general, suddenly. Its invasion is prompt, its duration variable, and its cure doubtful. Demonomania terminates in dementia. Convulsions, marasmus, scurvy, phthisis or a slow fever, bring to a close the life of this unfortunate class of our fellow beings. Demonomaniacs are emaciated, their complexion is sallow and sun-burnt, their physiognomy indicates disquietude, the look is suspicious, and the features of the face shrunken. They do not sleep, eat little, and often secretly. They walk much, and suffer from constipation. They are fond of solitude, experience pains in the head, chest, abdomen and limbs, and accuse the devil of it. They feel an internal fire which consumes them, and believe that they are in the flames of hell which they alone perceived. Their breath seems to be on fire. With groans they lament their fate, but never weep. They strive to injure those who surround them, and suffer from a thousand hallucinations, and even fury. The possessed exhale a very strong odor, which betrays, say they, the presence of the devil. This phenomenon is not rare in nervous maladies, either because the breath has become fetid, or because the transpiration has acquired an odor very much increased by the morbid character of the fluids. Does the fetor of the breath announce a threatening attack of convulsions, mania or hysteria? Women in a state of demonomania, experience a thousand hysterical symptoms. They believe that they are transported to the midnight assemblies of wizards, where they are witnesses of the strangest extravagances. They have intimate communications with the devil or his subordinates; after which, a collapse bringing an end to the attack, they find themselves again in the same place, from whence they believed they had been taken. Who does not see in this, the last stage of an attack of hysteria? Amidst the obscenities of these meetings, which we shall be cautious about describing,—who does not recognize the turpitude of an imagination, polluted by the vilest, most obscene and disgusting debauchery? who does not recognize a description of the most extravagant, shameful and ribald dreams? The frequent ecstasies which take place in nervous affections, partake of a sublime and contemplative character, if, during its waking hours, the soul is elevated to the contemplation of noble and divine objects. They are erotic, if the mind and heart lull themselves in reveries of love. They are obscene, if, when awake, one indulges in lascivious thoughts, and if the uterus, irritated and excited, gives place to illusions, which are regarded as diabolical practices.

The cases reported in the different articles of this work, establish the correctness of this view. Besides, they strikingly resemble the case of Angèle de Soligny, reported by Martin Del-Rio. Did not this female present all the features of nymphomania, provoked by widowhood, and a contemplative life carried to an extreme, and combated by religious principles? In the description of the nightly meetings of the witches, are united all those circumstances which are proper to excite the imagination. Assemblies, devoted to mysterious rites, have at all times been holden during the night. Night is most favorable to illusions and to fear. It presides over dreams. An uninhabited island, a rugged rock, a cavern surrounded by an ancient forest, an old and abandoned château, a cemetery, etc., such were the places of rendezvous. The adoration of the he-goat, dates back to the earliest period. It appertains to an ancient religious custom of the Egyptians, who offered, in Mendes, an infamous worship to the he-goat Hazazel. The ancients were in the habit of joining to prayers and invocations, the preparation of certain plants, and the immolation of certain animals, devoted to the infernal powers. Children also, were sacrificed. From the time of the introduction of christianity, sorcery allied itself to those notions of spirituality that prevailed. It borrowed from the christian worship, crosses, prayers and consecrated wafers; and profaned these sacred objects in a manner most revolting, in order to avenge the devil for his defeat. The sorcerers of Ireland, always recite the *Ave Maria* in their practices of sorcery. In Livonia, the grand talisman against sorcery consists in the following words; *Two eyes have regarded thee; three others can cast upon thee a favorable look, in the name of the Father, Son and Holy Ghost.*

Like all lypemaniacs, demonomaniacs suffer from hallucinations and illusions of the senses. Some think that they are the devil, others persuade themselves that they have the devil within them, who pinches, bites, rends and burns them. Some hear him speak, and his voice proceeds from the stomach, bowels or uterus. They converse with him, the devil recommending to them the commission of crimes, murders, acts of incendiarism and suicide. He provokes them to the most disgusting obscenities, and to blasphemies the most impious. He threatens and even *strikes* them, if they do not obey his orders. Many, who were retained in prison on account of their possession, assured those about them, that the devil had come thither to find them. Do we not see maniacs and melancholics, who converse with imaginary beings, who, they persuade themselves, are at their side, and were introduced by the chimney and window? The illusions of sight and touch, are here the same as with demonomaniacs. Some of the possessed or sorcerers, as a conveyance to their nightly assemblages, bestrode a broom. Others were mounted upon a he-goat, an ass, dog, etc. The latter, anointed the body with an ointment. The former had need only of their imaginations. All, without passing up the chimney, leaving their habitation, or even getting out of bed, reached the place of meeting, where they saw the devil; now, in the shape of a he-goat, a satyr or black cat; now, in that of a man, either black or white. Such are the disgusting reveries that have given rise to the belief in the existence of incubi and succubi. Some women, mostly hysterical, have seen the devil under the form of a young man, handsome, and well made. Doubtless libertines, abusing the weakness of some women, have borrowed from the devil his form and power. I once had in charge a maniac, who every night believed that he went to bed with his mistresses, and was accustomed to converse with them, assuming a different tone with each, and having reference to their respective dispositions and humor. There are many erotic lypemaniacs, who are convinced that they have had intimate relations with men, to whom they have scarcely addressed a word, but by whom their imagination has been taken.

Mad'lle de S., aged thirty-one years, of medium size, having black hair and eyebrows, a slender habit of body, and nervous temperament, together with a disposition disposed to melancholy, in company with her mother attends the botanical course of a celebrated professor. After a few lectures she persuades herself that she is pregnant by the professor, who is advanced in life, and to whom she has never spoken. Nothing dissuades her from this belief. She becomes much emaciated, loses her appetite, and is invincibly opposed to listening again to him who has made her a mother. The menses are suppressed, which is a new proof of pregnancy. The counsels of a tender and beloved mother, physicians and medicines, are all repulsed with obstinacy. She spends the eighth month in preparing child-bed linen. The ninth and tenth month pass without confinement. It does not take place, says the patient, because there are not colics and necessary pains. She stands much with naked feet, in order to provoke pains. She hears the father of her child, who exhorts her to patience, and encourages her to support the throes favorable to parturition. She sometimes utters cries, which are common to women at this period. In other respects, she is perfectly rational. I know well that I am like an insane person, she sometimes says, but it is certain that I am pregnant. She is committed to my care after suffering from this malady for eighteen months. She is very much emaciated and feeble, pulse frequent and small, skin dry and hot. She is sad, neither speaking nor moving; wishing neither to sit down during the day, nor to retire during the night. She also refuses all nourishment. I was enabled to overcome her unwillingness to take food, by effusions of cold water. But nothing triumphed over the convictions of this patient, who, some months after, went into the country to terminate her earthly pilgrimage.

The continual muttering of some of the possessed, has given rise to the belief that these unfortunate beings conversed with the devil in an unintelligible manner. We find this symptom existing in a great many melancholics, especially among those who have fallen into a state of dementia, and who stammer, in a low voice, words having no connection. The possessed, like all melancholics, beset by their own ideas, neglected their relatives, friends and interests. They were miserable and unfortunate; never improving, in a pecuniary respect, the condition of their family. They could no more do it, than deliver themselves from the demons and judges who were going to burn them. Improvidence, and incapacity for every kind of occupation, are the characteristics, not only of lypemania, but also of most of those passions which are intimately connected with it. The possessed were very obstinate in their belief, rarely betraying their adherence to it. Notwithstanding the severest punishments, in spite of the rack, which was most inhuman, the greater part remained attached to their notions, and obstinately refused to renounce their compact. The demon gave them this power and obstinacy. They were abandoned of God, who detested their abominations. This infatuation is characteristic of melancholy. Neither reasoning, privations, nor pain, can convince the lypemaniac. The stronger the efforts made to persuade him, the greater is his resistance, and the more powerfully does he withstand. Suspicion, fear and self-love fortify his convictions, which punishments only increase. I had in charge a young man who, deceived by an exaggerated notion of honor, refused all nourishment. After having exhausted all known means to overcome this resolution, I applied with much preparation, red hot irons upon different parts of his body, without overcoming his purpose. A surprise succeeds better. What can man not support, when sustained by a strongly excited imagination! The children of Sparta, lacerated by whips upon the altar of Diana, expired without uttering a complaint. A child at Lacedemon, having stolen a fox, concealed him beneath his tunic, and permitted his abdomen to be mangled by the teeth and claws of the animal, without manifesting the least pain, through fear of being discovered. To how great an extent does insensibility proceed in hysteria and convulsions!

The princess B., twenty seven-years of age, of a nervous temperament, a very lively imagination, a gay and mild disposition, had received a very excellent and liberal education, too strictly intellectual for a woman. Married when very young, she meets with great domestic trials, which repress her natural gayety, and render her melancholic. Missionaries go to St. Petersburg, and obtain permission to preach. Their sermons produce a strong impression upon the minds of the great ladies of that country. The imagination of the princess is not the last to become excited. See her now, an enthusiast, and uncertain whether she shall abandon the prevailing mode of worship. The sovereign, at first, expresses his dissatisfaction, and afterwards sends back the missionaries. Every one fears to incur the displeasure of a sovereign whom he loves. The princess, enfeebled by her sorrow, is easily subjugated by religious terrors, and the apprehension of a persecution. She becomes a lypemaniac, accuses herself of having committed crimes, and expresses a dread of being exposed to suffer martyrdom. Her aberration of mind increases, and one day, either to punish herself, or to test her courage, she places the middle finger of the right hand in the flame of a wax candle, and allows it to remain there so long, that it was necessary to remove its three phalanges, so deep had been the burn. At the expiration of four years, alternating between agitation and fury, composure and sadness, excitement and depression, the princess is brought to Paris and committed to my care. She was in a state of dementia complicated with paralysis, and attended with a disposition to transports of passion, and to strike when opposed. What could I do to overcome a disease like this? Her physical condition is improved, but reason was forever lost.

Punishments, invented by the most refined cruelty, could not draw tears from the eyes of the possessed when put to the torture. The demon, said they, dried up their source. Almost all lypemaniacs experience a desire to weep, without the ability to shed a tear, by whatever effort they may make. The sleep, into which some fell during the tortures of the rack, was the strongest proof of possession. They did not then know, that excessive pain produces an uncontrollable desire to sleep. They were accustomed to bind the limbs of the possessed before casting them into the water; and if they then swam upon it, they were regarded as possessed. Some hysterical women could not submerge themselves in the water, and floated when plunged into it. Those in favor of the punishment of the possessed, recommended that these unfortunates be interrogated, immediately after their arrest; because, so soon as they are taken, they think that they are forsaken by the devil, and confess every thing; whilst, if we allow them time to reflect, the devil comes and gives them instruction, (Del-Rio, Bodin, de l'Ancre). Who can forget the effects of a lively and vigorous impression, which always suspends the delirium for some moments, only to resume its power, so soon as the first effect of this moral commotion has ceased? Upon this phenomenon, reposes the most important therapeutic precept, for the treatment of the insane. Some of the possessed, unable to support the miseries they experienced, and incapable of resisting the varied solicitations which the devil made to them, pursued by remorse for crimes which they had committed, or with which they charged themselves, tormented by their thoughts, and tortured in a thousand ways, solicited death, prayed that the time of punishment might be hastened, threatened to destroy themselves, and marched gayly to the scaffold. Is not this symptom common to many melancholics, who prefer death a thousand times, to the disquietudes and anguish that torment, and the moral suffering which overwhelms them; an agony more intolerable than all the physical pains imaginable? Others on the contrary, persuaded that they could not die, (the devil having given them an assurance of it), went to their punishment with composure and tranquility; sometimes with disdain. This sense of security, which depended upon an illusion, a deceitful hope, was regarded as an incontestable proof of the presence of a demon. I have reported the cases of lypemaniacs, who were fully convinced that they could not die, and who were accustomed to enquire of me, what they should do, when left alone upon the earth. Convulsions existed in all times, because they depended upon the state of the organism, as well as the imagination. They complicate all the forms of mental alienation. Priestesses, sybils and pythonissæ fell into convulsions when the prophetic spirit took possession of them. The possessed were seized with convulsions when the delirium was very intense, and some became maniacs, *enraged*, and died. This termination, which is not rare in convulsive diseases, was regarded as the last effort of the devil, constrained to leave the body of the possessed person; the knaves took advantage of it, the better to deceive the ignorant. In reading the histories, reported by writers on demonology, and preserved in the accounts of the trials of the possessed, we learn that those contortions, convulsions, and great muscular contractions, referred to as efforts of the devil, are nothing more than those nervous symptoms, to which hysterical persons, hypochondriacs and epileptics, are all exposed. These convulsions did not deceive Pigrai when appointed to pronounce upon fourteen unfortunate persons, who had been condemned to the flames. He decided that hellebore should be given them. They did not triumph over the learned men who saw them at St. Medard, nor over the magistrate who caused them to cease at his will; notwithstanding, the murmur of certain rogues, who desired longer to abuse the public credulity.

From what precedes, we conclude:

1. That demonomania is a variety of religious melancholy.
2. That it recognizes as its remote cause, ignorance, prejudices and the feebleness and pusillanimity of the human mind.
3. That disquietude, fear and dread provoke it.
4. That the delirium, determinations and actions of demonomaniacs, depend upon, as their principal cause, false notions of religion, and a frightful depravation of morals.
5. That this disease has become more rare, since religious knowledge, a better education, and more general instruction, have more uniformly enlightened all classes of society.

We must signalize as one of the varieties of demonomania, that state in which some insane persons, stricken by the terrors of hell, believe that they are damned. These are persons whose minds are feeble, timid and fearful; whose hearts are upright and pure; whose convictions are profound, and who think that they have committed errors and crimes whose chastisement they cannot shun. Such are in a state of despair They are not, like demonomaniacs, actually in the power of the devil. They neither see nor feel the sulphureous flames which devour them.

Still they dread damnation, and are convinced that their career will terminate in hell. They impose upon themselves mortifications more or less extreme, as well as singular, in order to avoid their destiny. The history of all religions presents the cases of men who, fearful of the future, submit both their bodies and minds to the most cruel and inconceivable tortures; now, to secure the favors of heaven; and now, to disarm the celestial anger. A pusillanimous disposition, exaggeration, ignorance of the true principles of religion; the reading of books calculated to enslave the mind, the critical period, masturbation, and reverses of fortune; are the most frequent causes of this variety, which, in our day, is not so rare as demonomania, and does not spare, like it, the higher ranks of society. Demonomania furnishes the most striking proof of the strange opposition which exists between the ideas and determinations. The impulse to murder and suicide is very much to be feared among individuals, who stand in fear of eternal damnation. Sauvages, Forestus and Pinel, mention several cases of them. It is neither the spleen, nor disgust of life, which urges them on to suicide. It is neither the fright, which, depriving man of the faculty of reasoning, precipitates him upon the evil which he most fears. How happens it, said I to a young man, that you fear being damned, and yet wish, by taking your own life, to hasten on the period of eternal punishment, the very thought of which fills you with despair? This simple mode of reasoning he could not comprehend. Fear is a sentiment which is surmounted by a still stronger one. Persons who fear eternal damnation, are indescribably miserable. Solely occupied by their sufferings and actual torments, imagination represents this state of anguish as the greatest of evils; as greater than death itself. The evils which they dread, but do not feel, necessarily produce less effect upon them, than those which they endure. Future ills can be but imaginary, whilst actual ones are realities. Their intolerable position is frightful, and must be changed. Not having the courage to suffer, how should they have to hope? All is despair. This state of things must cease, cost what it may. The surest means of effecting it, is to cease to live. The resolution is taken,—reason wanders,—the future—and the punishments of hell, vanish. Delirium and despair direct the steel of the monomaniac, who commits self-murder.

Of all insane persons lypemaniacs are the most cruel. Not only do these wretched beings attempt their own destruction; but direct their deadly blows at the persons of their friends, relatives and children. A miserable being, after listening to a sermon, believing himself damned, goes home and destroys his children to preserve them from the same dreadful doom (Pinel). A young woman experiences certain domestic trials. She immediately persuades herself that she is lost, and for more than six months is haunted with the desire to destroy her children, to preserve them from the sufferings of a future state. When suffering from this frightful form of insanity, and, yielding to their blind fury, these wretched beings have executed their horrible purposes, they are never restored. Such is my experience. We are of the opinion that returning reason, bringing with it but too just reproaches, induces moral suffering, and gives rise to the most poignant regrets, which are shortly succeeded by the same torments and delirium. The treatment of demonomania is the same with that of lypemania, or melancholy with delirium. The pharmaceutic treatment, as well as the regimen, depend upon the knowledge of its causes. Albrecht tells us, that he cured a robust man, who for some years was regarded as possessed, by causing him to take wine, impregnated with emetic qualities, during alternate periods of fourteen days; at the fourth period his patient was cured.*

The moral means do not differ from those which are adapted to lypemania in general. The assistance of ministers of religion has rarely been followed with permanent success. A lady believed herself damned, and had recourse to several priests. A prelate, as respectable by his age as his virtues, went to her residence arrayed in his pontifical robes, received her confession, and lavished upon her religious consolations. The patient recovered her reason perfectly for a few hours; but on the following day, she relapsed into a state worse than her former one had been. However, I by no means think that such aid ought to be neglected. The consolations of religion, the presence and encouragements of a minister of the altar, by calling into exercise a degree of confidence on the part of the patient, may cause hope to spring up in his breast, and prove the commencement of a cure. We find several examples of cures among authors. Zacutus relates, that he restored to health a demonomaniac, by introducing into his chamber during the night, an individual in the guise of an angel, who announced to the patient that God had pardoned him. We can imagine, that success might attend the like efforts in similar cases. If the disease is not of long standing, if it is not complicated with organic lesions, with paralysis or

*Philosopical Decade, year iv.

scurvy, we may hope for a degree of success. Reil suggests a great number of means, but reduces all to this general principle: to make a vivid impression upon the imagination of the insane, in order to subjugate it, and afterwards to gain possession of their confidence and mind; or to combat a passion by a passion. To do this, an observing mind is necessary, and a thorough acquaintance with the management of the understanding and passions of men.

Connected with demonomania as a sub-variety, is Zoanthropy; a deplorable aberration of the mind, which perverts the instinct even, and persuades the lypemaniac that he is changed into a brute. This strange form of insanity has been observed from the highest antiquity; and was connected with the worship of the ancient pagans who sacrificed their animals to their gods. Lycanthropy was described by Ætius and the Arabians. It has been known since the fifteenth century, and they have given in France, to those afflicted with this disease, the appellation of wolf-men. These wretched beings fly from their fellow men, live in the woods, church-yards and ancient ruins, and wander, howling, about the country at night. They permit their beard and nails to grow, and thus become confirmed in their deplorable conviction, by seeing themselves covered with long hair, and armed with claws. Impelled by necessity or a cruel ferocity, they fall upon children, tear, slay and devour them. Roulet, at the end of the sixteenth century, was arrested as a wolf-man, and confessed, that with his brother and cousin, after having rubbed the body with an ointment, they were changed into wolves, and that they ran about the fields, and devoured children. Justice, more enlightened than in the preceding ages of the world, sent those unfortunate men to a hospital for the insane.

There have been lycanthropes who believed that they were transformed into dogs. These are called cynanthropes. A distinguished lord of the court of Louis XIV, experienced, at times, a disposition to bark, and was accustomed to put his head out of the window to satisfy this desire. Don Calmet tells us that in a convent in Germany, the nuns believed that they were changed into cats, and that, at a certain hour of the day, they were accustomed to run all about the convent, striving to outdo each other in mewing. We find, even in our days, insane persons who, no longer believing in the power of the devil over matter, still believe *in destiny*; and persuade themselves that it imposes upon them all the pains they suffer; that they are objects of horror, and ought to be removed from the world. This unfortunate caprice manifests itself in the country. We have at Charenton a young man from the mountains of Limousin, of a bilious-sanguine temperament, slender and emaciated in his habit, with black hair and eyes, and a pale complexion, who has a *dracq* in his abdomen. The dracq, or destiny, sometimes enters his head, tortures him in a thousand ways during the day, and particularly in the night, addresses and threatens him. If I ask this unfortunate young man what this dracq may be, "I know nothing about it," he replies, "but it is a destiny that has been imposed upon me, and every thing has been done to deliver me from it, but without success." Other lypemaniacs are convinced that they have no head, that they have one of glass or of a bird, that an enormous excrescence depends from the nose, and that their body is of butter, their limbs of wax or of glass. We must also speak again of that singular perversion, which persuades a young woman at Charenton that she no longer has a body, and who is constantly going about, like a person who has lost his way, seeking for her body. She calls upon us for it, during a visit, and repeats incessantly, "I have no longer a body,—what will become of me! give me my body." Hippocrates understood the cause of the disease of the Scythians, which sometimes appears in our days, from different influences.

Mad'e M., a widow, experienced, after the death of her husband, very great trials, together with the loss of her fortune. She has an attack of mania, makes attempts to commit suicide, and is sent to the Salpêtrière. She was small in stature, very much emaciated, much agitated, constantly talking, assuring us and repeating with transports of emotion, that she was not a woman, but a man. If any one, in speaking to her, addresses her with the appellation of Madame, she immediately becomes more agitated, utters abusive language, or gives herself up to acts of violence. M. Pussin, then inspector in the direction of that department of the hospital devoted to insane women, engaged with M. Pinel to procure the dress of a man for this female. She attired herself in it with transports of joy, and walked about among her companions with a sort of ostentation. She was more composed and tranquil, and talked much less, but was excited to fury, if not addressed by the title of Monsieur instead of Madame. Her strength gradually gave way, and she entered the infirmary in the month of November, 1802, having a copious diarrhœa, and being exceedingly weak. She rejected baths, ptisans, and the potions that were prescribed for her. At length, she became unwilling to take any thing, and died, aged sixty-eight years, her delirium remaining unchanged to the last days of her life.

At the post-mortem examination, I found the external vessels of the cranium gorged with blood. The cerebral substance presented nothing remarkable, except numerous bloody points when it was divided by slices. The lateral ventricles contained each about two ounces of serum. The mucous membrane of the stomach, in its small curvature, presented an ulcer of about four inches in circumference, its surface being covered with granulations, and of a grayish aspect. Near the pylorus, there was a species of polypus, extremely soft, and large at its base, projecting about an inch, and having a brown color. Traces of inflammation were noticed upon the mucous membrane of the stomach, cecum, colon and rectum; and at some points this membrane was destroyed. The gall bladder contained bile of a deep green color, inspissated, and mingled with small concretions.

I had in charge, many years since, a man twenty-six years of age, of a noble stature, large size, and genteel figure, who, in his earliest youth, was very fond of dressing himself in women's clothes. Admitted into the highest circles, if a comedy was performed, he always chose the part of a female. At length, in consequence of a trifling opposition, he persuaded himself that he was a woman, and sought to convince every body of it, even the members of his family. Several times did he, while at home, divest himself of all his clothes, array himself with the head-dress and costume of a nymph, and, thus attired, wished to walk abroad in the streets. When committed to my care, aside from this notion, he was not irrational. He was however, constantly occupied in curling his hair, in admiring himself in the glass, and with his dressing gowns, used every effort to render his costume as similar as possible to that of a woman. He was accustomed, also, to imitate their step when walking. One day while walking with him in the garden, I raised the lappet of his riding coat, which he had carefully arranged, when immediately he takes one step backward, and treats me in an impertinent and lewd manner. No reasoning, attention nor regimen, were successful in restoring this unfortunate man to the use of his reason.

12

Cinematic Neurosis Following "The Exorcist"

Report of Four Cases

JAMES C. BOZZUTO, *M.D.*[1]

Following the distribution and release of the movie, "The Exorcist," much publicity concerning the psychiatric hazards of the film were reported. Numerous cases of traumatic neurosis and even psychosis were supposedly noted. This report confirms the hypothesis that traumatic "cinema neurosis" can be precipitated by viewing the movie in previously unidentified psychiatric patients. The paper will examine an early reported case by Freud, investigate some underlying psychological principles in the book, and then report on the presentation and treatment of four cases.

This movie seems to be directly related to traumatic neurosis in susceptible people. Classical symptoms and disability were observed following viewing the movie. There are ele-

[1]Cincinnati General Hospital, Ohio.

Reprinted with permission from *The Journal of Nervous and Mental Disease*, 1975, vol. 161, 43–48.

> ments in the movie, such as possession with resultant loss of impulse control, that are likely to threaten people with similar problems, and to exceed their "stimulus barrier." Suggested treatment recommends brief, early access treatment, using the movie to help each patient to explore where he identified and to understand some of his ambivalent conflicts with either parents or spouse.

Of all of the writings of Freud, his paper, "A Seventeenth-Century Demonological Neurosis" (3), published in 1922, ranks as one of the least read and least well known. The possession of Christoph Haizmann is a case report from a number of sources, including the work of a clerical compiler, the artist's own diary, and copies of his artistic productions portraying his possession and exorcism. In short, the artist suffered a severe depression following the death of his father. He had "become low-spirited, was unable or unwilling to work properly and was worried about making a livelihood; that is to say he was suffering from melancholic depression with an inhibition in his work . . ." (3, p. 80). He thereupon was approached by the Devil who offered to relieve his sufferings for the promise of support and a blood pact for the next 9 years. The artist agreed, and signed the pact to be freed from his depression. The depression was then alleviated for the next 9 years, and was only reported because he sought an exorcism at the end of the pact.

Freud is quite clear and succinct that the Devil in this case represented "bad or reprehensible wishes, derivatives of instinctual impulses that have been repudiated and repressed" (3, p. 72), and that the artist chose the Devil as a father substitute for the death of his real father. The retention of the Devil today would be more clearly understood as the retention of a part object in the face of loss, as a partial solution to that loss.

Following the distribution and release of the movie, "The Exorcist," numerous cases of traumatic neurosis and even psychosis were supposedly noted (2, 6, 7). The parallels between Freud's case and the book, *The Exorcist* by William Peter Blatty (1) are striking. The story involves a 13-year-old girl who, in the movie, is noted to be suffering some depression, following the divorce and separation from her biological father who fails to call her on her birthday. We are not presented with any actual clinical evidence into her depression but are alerted that she views her potential stepfather with contempt, and in one of the first indications of possession, she predicts his death and seems somehow involved in his demise. The story continues with her increasing possession by demonological forces, rapidly developing impulses of rage and aggressions, directed at her mother and eventually at the two priests who are called in to perform the exorcism.

The main psychological themes in both histories seem to be the loss of a parent, depression, and some psychological attempt at restitution by retention of part objects in the form of the Devil. The question of whether this theme itself—possession following loss—is sufficient to explain the incidence of traumatic neurosis following the movie or whether the sheer brutality and violence can account for it, will be explained in more detail following the case reports.

Also examined will be the prior knowledge or lack of it that patients had concerning the film and its contents, some of their religious background, who attended the film with the patients, and how they spent their time afterward, for we feel that these may be important variables. Also, the severity of neurosis and the presenting symptoms will be examined.

CASE REPORTS

Case 1.

Norman N. was an 18-year-old white male who presented to the emergency room with the complaint that for the past 3 weeks since he had seen the movie, "The Exorcist," he had been unable to take his mind off of it. Six months prior to this, he had joined the Marines to avoid a minor police charge, and had been stationed 2000 miles from home. He was the only adopted child of an elderly religious couple who felt quite concerned about him. While in the service, he had become "homesick" and lonely, and had sought out a Bible study group who served free food to service men. He became interested in God and "asked God into my heart" approximately 2 weeks before he returned home for his first leave. He described this as a conversion, "that I had felt God came into me" and felt euphoric until the movie.

When he returned home for the first time, a group of friends asked him to go to a late night movie. He had no prior knowledge of what to expect, felt "shaky and unsure" during the movie, returned home, noted the similarity of his bed to that in the movie, and was unable to sleep. He was found at 4 or 5 a.m. by his father, clutching a Bible in the dark. His manifest fear was that the Devil could possess him. After the first evening, he continued to be unable to sleep for the next 3 or 4 nights, heard "creaky noises" in the evening, noted decreased appetite, irritability, and inability to remove the scenes from his mind. After 3 days, he left home, and began drinking and abusing multiple drugs to obliterate all memory of the movie. This had failed and he returned home after 2 weeks with the original symptoms.

He felt he was in danger of possession for all of the bad things he had done in his life, felt the only way one could be saved was to "take God into your heart, he's your father and if you are his son he will take care of you." His father brought him to the emergency room.

Case 2.

James V., a 23-year-old white male, was referred by a priest to the psychiatric outpatient clinic 1 month after viewing the movie. Since that time, he had been unable to sleep, had decreased appetite, irritability, paranoia, decreased sexual functioning, and was unable to remain alone for any period of time. He knew quite a bit about the movie before he had seen it, his wife having read parts of the book extensively to him. He saw the film with her, felt relatively uncomfortable during the movie, but that evening talked with his wife and didn't note any disturbance. The next evening his wife stayed out late and left him with their 4-year-old daughter. As the evening progressed, he became more upset, brought his daughter into the same room and felt he was becoming possessed. He was simultaneously preoccupied with thoughts of impending injury or accidental death of his wife. He also had fears that she might have been with another man. When she returned at 4 a.m. he was relieved, and said nothing.

He had a vacation the following week, but from that night on, he complained of insomnia, had persistent magical dreams of the Devil, was unable to stay alone, and tended to "misinterpret sounds." He stated "I entertained the idea I could be guilty about something."

The patient was the oldest of two siblings, whose mother moved quite a bit. His father was divorced when the patient was 2 and from then on he lived mainly in the home of his maternal grandparents, which "was the only secure place, the only place I could call home."

He had been married for 5 years and complained that both he and his wife were disappointed in the marriage. He was upset at her for not caring for him and the household, while she stated that he was dull, uninteresting, and tended to stay at home. He was unable to express any anger at his wife for fear of losing control, although he had hit her only once in 5 years.

He returned to work after 1 week as a stockboy, but felt he would meet the Devil around any corner, became moderately paranoid, and finally sought the advice of a priest who referred him.

Case 3.

Martha B., a 22-year-old white female, called the Psychiatric Clinic stating that she had been unable to sleep for approximately 1 week after viewing the movie "The Exorcist." For the previous 7 days, Ms. B. had been unable to sleep, was having difficulties with anxiety reactions in which she became sweaty, had abdominal cramps, hyperventilated, and was afraid that someone was after her or she was going to die.

She had talked with people who had been frightened by the movie before she saw it, thought she could view it without being bothered, and went with her boyfriend. She remembered being concerned with the young priest and wondering if he had gone to Hell. That night she couldn't sleep, felt "so bad I was considering hospitalization, was in panic and even contemplated suicide." She stated that it was better during the day and work helped but that during the evening she became "sensitive to sounds," became irritable both at work and with her boyfriend. She explained that she was preoccupied with "the Devil aspect" and the fact that evil forces seemed to predominate. She was especially aware of the priest's difficulty with his mother, and associated that to remembering wishing her mother would die when she was age 13. That weekend her mother had a stroke and the patient spent the next 4 years caring for her.

The patient was an only child of strict religious Catholic parents. As noted, she remembered being angry at her mother when she was 13 and wished her dead, and that weekend she had suffered a severe stroke. Her parents insisted that she attend all girls Catholic grade and high schools. After 1 year of college, she left home and went to a state university to become an occupational therapist against her parents' wishes. For the past 3 months she had been living with a boyfriend and having sexual relations, both of which were against her parents' wishes but known to them. She felt the movie had "opened up lots of feelings about her parents." She also felt she had considerable amounts of guilt and was "punishing herself by now living with this man." She resented her Catholic background, felt leaving the church was like leaving her parents, and that the movie had brought up guilt of punishment for bad feelings toward her parents. She found herself "furious at her loss at work and had feelings of killing all older people or parental figures," and was afraid of losing control, becoming enraged and hysterical.

Case 4.

Mr. Lyle H. was a 24-year-old black male who initially came to the emergency room for three visits approximately 1 month after seeing "The Exorcist." At that time, he complained of flashbacks and of getting "nervous," especially with his two children and his wife; he was frightened that his 5-year-old daughter was possessed, had insomnia, and felt that certain people "looked strange." He was given Valium and referred to the Psychiatric Clinic. After being contacted for his first interview, he was fearful of coming for he felt that the therapist may have been involved with the Devil.

The patient stated that he knew little about the movie, but had seen it discussed on a T.V. talk show before. He went with his wife and another couple. He was so upset during the movie that he had to walk out, and afterward he was frightened, feeling that the Devil "would come." He had immediate insomnia, 15-pound weight loss over the past month, and numerous nightmares of vampires chasing a woman with himself interfering. He could not look people directly in the eye for fear he might imagine them to be devils.

The patient was the youngest of six siblings and presently lived in an apartment with his wife and two children in the same building that his parents own. He described his marriage as good but that because of his low income and inability to buy a car or rent his own apartment he and wife argued considerably. She wised to return to work and buy a car but he felt, "I like to be the boss in my own home." In the previous few months, she had left the family because of financial arguments but had always returned. He described himself as unable to express his own anger and always wanting to please her, but being in conflict with being his own boss. He was afraid of expressing his feeling for fear of either losing her or hurting her feelings.

Also, since seeing the movie, he complained of a stiff neck which he related to an identification with the girl in the movie. He was afraid to use a razor that his brother-in-law had given him because it might be stolen and it would imply he had done something wrong and would therefore be like the Devil.

RESULTS

All four patients presented remarkably similar symptoms which, in all cases, began the same evening that they viewed the movie or within 1 day. The classical symptoms of insomnia, excitability, hyperactivity, irritability, and decreased appetite were present in all four, and other symptoms of decreased sexual functioning, impending loss of impulse control, paranoia, and drug and alcohol abuse were present in others. Two of the four cases initiated psychiatric care within 1 week, while the other two waited 2 to 3 weeks. Only one patient had a prior psychiatric history and that had been for eight visits at a university health clinic.

Extensive prior knowledge of the film was present in three of the four and did not seem to offer protection from symptoms. Religion was an important part of the family structure of three of the four patients, and seemed very significant to two, Martha B. and Norman N. Brief active psychotherapy was the treatment in all cases, and in only one was psychoactive medication given (diazepam, Lyle H.). All responded within three to seven hourly sessions, and were relatively free of disturbing symptoms and able to return to their prior levels of functioning with the termination of therapy. Although follow-up was offered, there was none after 6 months (see Table 1).

DISCUSSION

All cases suffered moderate to severe disorganization after viewing the movie. The movie was the traumatic event in that three of the four had no prior psychiatric history, all four developed disturbing symptoms within 1 day of seeing the movie, and all four identified the movie as the precipitating event. In the earliest formulation of trauma, Freud suggested that the term applies to "an experience which within a short

TABLE 1
Summary of Patients

PATIENT	AGE	RELIGION	SYMPTOMS	ONSET OF SYMPTOMS	SOUGHT TREATMENT	TREATMENT: NO. OF SESSIONS	PREVIOUS TREATMENT
1. Norman N.	18-year-old white male	Protestant	Insomnia, appetite loss, scared, drug and alcohol abuse, agitation, hyperexcitability	Same day	1 month	3	0
2. James V.	23-year-old white male	Protestant	Insomnia, appetite loss, irritability, unable to work, decreased sexual functioning, paranoia	1 day later	3 weeks	3	0
3. Martha B.	22-year-old white female	Catholic	Insomnia, irritability, suicidal impulses, hostile rage at parental figures	Same night	1 week	7	8
4. Lyle H.	24-year-old black male	Protestant	Insomnia, nightmares, difficulty working, somatic identification, ideas of reference	Same night	1 to 2 weeks	6	0

period of time presents the mind with an increase of stimulus too powerful to be dealt with or worked off in the usual way" (4, p. 11), and this constituted the stimulus barrier concept of trauma. Overwhelming this barrier results in defects in "affect discharge leaving the mind still hypersensitive to even minor stimuli, *i.e.*, excitations that would not have disturbed personality equilibrium prior to trauma" (8, p. 43).

Using this model, the movie was a precipitant that exceeded the stimulus barrier in all four cases and presented each with disturbing and classical symptoms. The question of exactly what was traumatic for each patient was not entirely clear. Each, however, at the time of viewing the film, had potential problems with loss either of parent or spouse, and had marked ambivalence to that person. The common element in the movie that seemed threatening to all was the loss of impulse control to an ambivalently cathected person. However, only one patient presented this as an initial complaint, but all eventually acknowledged this as the threat.

The movie thus forced them to experience anger and hostility (repressed in three or four) at this ambivalently cathected object and resulted in these fears of identification with the Devil, or in concerns over possession, and all four expressed intense feelings of guilt for their aggressive feelings.

Norman N. had just returned home from over 6 months of separation from his parents whom he considered strict and harsh. He described being lost and taking God into his heart only 2 weeks before the movie. He admitted uncontrollable aggressive impulses toward his parents, and at one point recollected hitting his mother in the back when he was 4, following her recovery from back surgery. His reaction to the movie was intense guilt and fear that he would become like Regan. The other two men had considerable difficulty with their wives preceding the movie and seemed unable to express their anger. Only the visualization of their actual impulses precipitated acute panic and disorganization.

Finally the woman, Martha, acknowledged intense rage at her parents at the time before the movie, and was actually engaged in behavior which did enrage her parents. She had also had feelings of wishing her mother dead from which she suffered recurrent guilt.

It was felt that each patient had a predisposition for trauma, especially trauma that was uncontrolled and directed toward "close" relationships. The movie was traumatic therefore not because of its use of violence, or aggression, but because it portrayed uncontrollable forces within the person, which could be unleashed by outside forces over which one had no control.

This, then, formed the basis of therapeutic intervention. Each patient varied in his degree of awareness of direct hostile feelings toward his spouse or parent. Interpretation was made first on an interpersonal level then on an intrapsychic level. The ambivalence of the patient's relationships was explored in each case with direct reference to the movie and raised questions about their own aggressiveness. The movie was used therapeutically as a metaphor by the therapist to help each to understand what was particularly uncomfortable about the movie and why he became symptomatic after seeing it. In all cases, brief treatment varying from three to seven hourly sessions seemed sufficient.

The other interesting aspect of this movie was that trauma following cinema is relatively unreported. There seems to be no literature on this subject, and when this movie was presented before a large psychiatric audience, only one therapist had remembered a case precipitated by Alfred Hitchcock's "Psycho." The author feels that perhaps cases do arise, but usually with mild symptomatology, and the patients do not seek treatment. There is some evidence that certain sensory modalities, *i.e.*, sight, are more susceptible to traumatic involvement, and this may be an element for future study. "Sensory modalities at birth and early in life . . . that can be stimulated but cannot adequately respond to the stimulus are possibly more susceptible to traumatic involvement" (5, p. 567). Although one patient did walk out of the movie, the others did not, and this did not seem to diminish his response.

It is anticipated that with further exploration by the film industry into the areas of the macabre and occult, more cases will be identified.

REFERENCES

1. Blatty, W. P. *The Exorcist*. Bantam Books, New York, 1972.
2. Exorcist fever. Time, *103*: (No. 6) 53, 1974.
3. Freud, S. A seventeenth-century demonological neurosis. In Strachey, J. *The Complete Psychological Works of Sigmund Freud*, Vol. 19, pp. 67–105. Hogarth Press, London, 1961.
4. Furst, S. *Psychic Trauma*, p. 11. Basic Books, New York, 1967.
5. Murphy, W. F. Character, trauma, and sensory perception. Int. J. Psychoanal., *39*: 555–568, 1958.

6. The Devil and Dr. Schlan. Med. World News, *15*: (No. 7) 5, 1974.
7. "The Exorcist" haunts M. D.'s at Georgetown. Am. Med. News, *17*: (No. 9) 14, 1974.
8. Titchener, J. L., and Ross, D. W. Acute or chronic stress as determinants of behavior, character, and neurosis. In Arieti, S., and Brody, E. B. *American Handbook of Psychiatry, III*, pp. 43–44. Basic Books, New York, 1974.

13

Cacodemonomania and Exorcism in Children

ERIC SCHENDEL, *M.D.*[1]
RONALD-FREDERIC C. KOURANY, *M.D.*[2]

ABSTRACT

Despite its popularity in the lay media, alleged possession of children by demons has received scant attention in the scientific literature. Five cases are presented. This phenomenon probably represents a variant of *folie à deux*. A religious consultant may advantageously be included as a member of the treatment team.

Cacodemonomania is the delusion of being possessed by a demon.[1] Although the occult has attracted sporadic interest in the medical literature, reports on the subject of exorcism of children are rare, despite its popularity in the lay media. Little is known of the psychologic impact on children of the accusation that they are demon-possessed. We review the recent psychiatric literature on demonology and present 5 cases of cacodemonomania involving children. A psychodynamic

[1,2]Vanderbilt University Medical Center, Nashville, Tennessee.

Reprinted with permission from *Journal of Clinical Psychiatry*, 1980, vol. 41, 119–123.

explanation of the delusion is proposed and some suggestions on management offered.

LITERATURE REVIEW

Studies of the occult go back to antiquity. By advocating a more enlightened approach to the insane than pyrotherapy, Johannes Wiero's[2] sixteenth century treatise *De Praestigiis Daemonum Et Incantationibus Ac Veneficiis* stands as a landmark in the history of western medicine.[3–5] Freud[6] provided a psychoanalytic foundation for understanding the occult when he observed that the "states of possession correspond to our neuroses . . . the demons are bad or reprehensible wishes, derivatives of instinctual impulses that have been repudiated and repressed."

After reviewing the literature, Yap[7] in 1960 examined 66 Hong Kong cases of cacodemonomania. He found that this delusion was more prevalent in divorced women or widows who were illiterate or from a low socioeconomic background. Nearly half of his cases were hysterical and almost a quarter schizophrenic. Ludwig[8–9] pointed out that belief in witchcraft can be cultural and asserted that it may be considered pathological only when maladaptive. He added that belief in witchcraft and demons was a defense mechanism that permitted the projection of unacceptable feelings and wishes onto a scapegoat. Leininger[10] also noted a cultural milieu that facilitated the projection of familial conflicts onto an outside group of witches who were felt to be responsible for the bewitchment of the victimized family member. A recent editorial[11] on exorcism inspired several letters to the editor[12–13] including one by Greenson[12] who suggested that the belief in possession represents an attempt to deny responsibility for "internal devilishness" through externalization; the ritual of exorcism then becomes appealing because it confirms the sense of being an innocent victim.

In the early 1970's *The Exorcist* heightened public interest in the occult and Bozzuto[14] presented 4 cases of traumatic neurosis that developed after viewing the film, which, he stated, mobilized hostility toward an ambivalently cathected object and resulted in a fear of identification with the devil. In 1975 Kiraly[15] published a case study of cacodemonomania presenting as *folie à deux*. The primary partner was an 18 year-old dependent schizophrenic girl who used the delusion as a paranoid defense against the hostility she felt toward her hysterical mother who accepted the delusion in order to maintain their relationship. Henderson[16] also drew on the popular literature, utilizing the novel *Dracula* as the framework for elaborating on object relations theory. He compared the persecuting supernatural forces to internalized bad objects and asserted that the interest in possession and exorcism was an advance in the public understanding of mental disorders, because this religious view of emotional distress, unlike the medical paradigm, placed the conflict inside the psyche. Spiegel and Fink,[17] in the context of a discussion of hypnosis and hysterical psychosis, presented a 15 year-old boy who believed he was possessed by "demons of Satan." They suggested that this delusion was a hysterical defense against his incestuous attraction to an older sister and his resentment against his family's religiosity.

Several authors have described how they incorporated their patients' beliefs into their therapeutic approaches. Citing an earlier article by McAll,[18] MacKarness[19] advocated exorcism for intractable cases of "demonosis." Casper and Philippus[20] used white magic in the form of suggestion and colorful low-dose doxepin tablets to treat the embrujada (bewitchment) syndrome among Mexican-Americans, most of whom diagnostically were anxious depressives. Cappannari et al[21] described a case of hexing that complicated the medical management of a 19 year-old woman with regional enteritis; she apparently lost her will to live until an exorcism was performed under psychiatric auspices by a fundamentalist minister. On the other hand, Lister[22] commented on a bizarre case in England where an attempted exorcism by a religious group delayed psychiatric intervention and resulted in uxoricide.

Other authors have recently examined the possession-exorcism theme.[23–43] Except for Israel and North[31] who presented a 5 year-old boy fatally abused by his parents because they believed he was possessed, and Teoh and Dass[39] who presented an 18 year-old Indian youth from Malaysia, none of these authors specifically discussed cacodemonomania in children. Five such cases have been culled from our mental health clinic population.

CASE HISTORIES

Case 1.

An 11-year-old boy was brought to the clinic by his mother because of difficulties with authority, school problems, rebelliousness and poor peer and sibling relationships of at least 1 year's duration.

His parents divorced when he was 5 years old after multiple separations. Contacts with his natural father were infrequent. The mother displayed considerable ambivalence toward her son. The family was Catholic but at one point the mother placed the boy in a Baptist minister's home, much to his disgust. During the evaluation she reported that following an accident in Israel when he was 7, his legs began to grow unequally. An American couple, who were faith healers, prayed for the boy in front of both mother and child, and "his short leg grew out" before their eyes. Since then the mother believed she was "gifted" at spiritual healing and specialized in healing legs.

When the boy was 10 his mother became involved in a religious group and sought counselling from an elder because of the boy's behavioral problems. The elder quoted scripture to him, "saved him" and had him promise to be obedient. When his acting out continued the elder suggested he was possessed by evil spirits and recommended an exorcism to be performed by himself and another elder. An attempt at exorcism was reportedly made and, according to the mother, the boy went totally "berserk" during the ritual and ran away. At a later date she denied that the exorcism was actually carried out but continued to speculate that her son's behavior might be due to demonic possession.

Mental status examination revealed a well developed, appropriately dressed, white boy who was alert and oriented. His speech was normal and there was no evidence of a thought disorder. He was friendly, well-behaved in the office, and engaging. His affect was appropriate but with a suggestion of depression and low self-esteem which he defended against with denial.

A diagnosis of adjustment reaction, depressive type was made and he was offered outpatient psychotherapy. The patient left town with his mother, however, after 9 sessions.

Case 2.

A 7 year old boy was admitted to the Child Psychiatry inpatient unit because of fighting, poor peer relations, and aggressiveness toward his mother.

The parents divorced when he was less than a year old. The mother remarried and was having multiple marital and psychiatric problems. She reported that the patient's behavioral problems had become so bad that she tried "everything" to correct him but to no avail. Among those unsuccessful attempts she listed spanking, arguing, and punishing. (Child abuse was suspected, as the child had been brought to the Emergency Room with a broken clavicle and multiple bruises). About 1 month prior to admission she was told, and quickly believed, by her fellow Church of God members, that "demons have taken possession" of the boy and that they needed to be driven out. A church service was organized and the members of the congregation all prayed together and "drove the demons out of him." The boy was reported to have been "flung across the room by some force" when this happened. This "force" left a "mark" on his face. The boy mentioned that he "was glad that the demons were gone" and "saw angels after they left." Worsening of his behavioral problems ultimately led to his psychiatric hospitalization.

The mental status examination revealed an alert, oriented and well developed white boy. He was verbal and cooperative. He had a wide range of affect. He had poor impulse control, difficulties talking about his relationship with his mother, and was confused about the chaotic home environment. There was no evidence of a thought disorder. His intelligence was within normal range and there was no evidence of organic impairment.

The diagnosis of severe anxiety reaction was considered. Some improvement during hospitalization was noted. He was discharged against medical advice on his mother's insistence and the State Department of Human Services was notified of suspected abuse.

Case 3.

An 11-year-old girl from a small rural community in Mississippi was admitted to the Child Psychiatry inpatient unit because of headaches, violent outbursts and poor peer relations. On one occasion she swung her small nephew by his feet and banged his head on the ground. On another occasion she stuck a thorn in her mother's leg. The patient stated that she was aware of what she was doing during these "spells" but could not control her body and that "someone else" was responsible. Her grandparents and mother decided she was possessed by the devil; she agreed.

Her parents divorced when she was less than 2 years old and her mother later remarried. Contact with the natural father was sporadic, then lost. The family religious background was fundamentalist, Church of Christ and Pentecostal. When the "family doctor could not find anything wrong" with her and after it was agreed that she was possessed by the devil, she was taken to a Pentecostal Church where she was prayed over for 3 consecutive nights so that she could be "healed" and "regain her faith." Afterwards she reported she felt better for a few days. When she started to have her spells again, she was brought to the Emergency Room and subsequently admitted to the hospital.

The mental status examination revealed a well developed white girl, appropriately dressed and groomed, who appeared older than her stated age and presented in a seductive manner. There was no unusual motor activity. She was soft-spoken and articulate. She talked about "spots before her eyes." Her affect was bland and indifferent. She was alert, oriented and appeared to be of above average intelligence. There was no evidence of a thought disorder.

Medical and neurological evaluations were negative and a tentative diagnosis of conversion reaction was made. She improved rapidly but was discharged against medical advice upon her mother's insistence.

Case 4.

A 17 year-old-girl was brought to the clinic because she believed she was possessed by the devil and was seeing the spirit of her dead mother. She also reported hearing and seeing other people and objects and was afraid of being followed and poisoned. The onset of these symptoms dated back at least 3 years with a gradual worsening.

The history revealed that the patient's mother, who had been a prostitute, was murdered when the patient was 12. She lived for a while with her maternal grandparents where she was molested, raped and involved in incestuous relationships with her uncle and cousin. Although healing or exorcism was denied, the patient's extended family was reported to be superstitious and "believed" in supernatural phenomena including curses, voodoo and witchcraft.

Mental status examination revealed an alert, oriented and well developed black teenager with a flat affect, delusions of influence and reference, thought insertion, thought broadcasting, and concrete thinking. She also had auditory and visual hallucinations. There was no evidence of organicity and her intellect was in the low normal range.

A diagnosis of paranoid schizophrenia was made and thioridazine was begun but she did not keep her follow-up appointment.

Case 5.

A 13-year old boy was admitted to the Child Psychiatry inpatient unit because of sleeping difficulties, withdrawal and bizarre behavior. He claimed to be able to talk to demons. They had "entered" his body 2 years earlier, but he "did not mind it then." Two months prior to admission they refused his attempt to "expel" them and he started feeling subject to their whims and wishes and felt compelled to smash glasses, tear things apart and fight with his brother. He claimed to be able to engage in astral projection (letting his soul leave his body to travel). He talked of using his demons to do "bad things" to people and "good things" for himself.

He was living with his schizophrenic mother and stepfather. His parents divorced when he was 4. His family was Baptist but expressed interest in witchcraft, black magic, mind reading, and telepathy. There was much conversation about demons and spirits. Religious intervention and healing were considered but never attempted.

Mental status examination revealed a well developed white male who was alert and oriented. He had auditory and visual hallucinations and grandiose delusions of reference and influence. He was withdrawn and aloof, sometimes condescending. His affect was flat. His intelligence was within the normal range.

Neurologic work-up was negative and a diagnosis of schizophrenia was made. He was started on thioridazine in the hospital but was discharged against medical advice after admission at his mother's insistence.

DISCUSSION

Several characteristics are common to these case histories. All the children had suffered the loss of 1 of their natural parents; 4 demonstrated aggressive acting out; and all 5 families terminated treatment prematurely, although 1 accepted referral to mental health professionals in another city.

Freud[6] felt his patient used the devil as a replacement for his dead father. Commenting on this and the fact that the book *The Exorcist* involves possession of a girl who has lost her father, Bozzuto[14] suggested that the belief one is possessed represents the retention of a part object as a defense against loss. This interpretation could apply to all 5 of our cases, since all 5 had lost 1 parent by death or divorce.

In at least 3 of our cases the belief in demon possession was initiated by someone other than the child, either a family member or a religious figure. The other 2 families were heavily invested in the occult. The defense of cacodemonomania may thus be primarily a manifestation of parental pathology. It would appear to be a shared delusion, a form of *folie à deux*. A modification of the dynamics suggested by Pulver and Brunt[44] and elaborated on by Kiraly[15] offers an explanation of what may be going on. They suggested that in a *folie à deux* the primary dependent partner feels increasingly taken advantage of and becomes progressively angrier at the other. Because of his dependency he cannot express his hostility directly but instead projects it onto an outsider. When the secondary partner initially refuses to accept the paranoid delusion, the primary partner's accusations "begin to shift toward the secondary partner, who finds this more direct hostility extremely anxiety provoking. . . . A point is reached where the tension becomes intolerable, and the secondary partner accepts the delusions. By deflecting his partner's hostility away from himself and reestablishing the projective defense, the secondary partner can now . . . ease his guilt, and express his own anger at the primary partner in projected form."[44]

In the case of children who are believed to be demon-possessed by their parents, it is our suggestion that the second portion of this dynamic process occurs. The primary dependent partner is the child who reacts to the loss of 1 parent and the ambivalence of the other with increasing hostility. This hostility mobilizes anxiety and guilt in the parent. To reduce the anxiety and guilt, the parent accepts the proposition, usually suggested by a third party, that the child is possessed. It is easier to believe that the anger comes from a demon than from one's own child. The child in turn finds that the delusion offers him a chance to reduce his own anxiety by resolving the conflict between his hostility and his dependency needs.

All our families terminated treatment prematurely. A reluctance to accept medical assistance by those who feel victimized by the occult was also noted by Leininger,[10] who wrote that 2 of her 6 families had earlier sought psychiatric assistance. It would appear that major cultural differences combine with the dynamics of the individual case to make conventional psychiatry unacceptable to these people.

By working within the cultural belief system of distressed individuals it has been possible to provide them assistance. Leininger[10] succeeded by providing family therapy in a supportive environment where her families could ventilate their anger and distrust toward each other and the hostile outside world. Spiegel's[17] patient was taught, through hypnosis, how to control his episodes of "possession." The young woman described in Cappannari[21] was able to obtain relief through an exorcism prescribed by the psychiatric consultant and performed by a Baptist minister.

Certainly we are not advocating exorcism for every patient who claims to be possessed; the long-term ramifications of such a ritual, particularly in highly impressionable children, are unknown. However, an attempt to bridge the cultural gap would appear to be in order. Child psychiatry relies heavily on a team approach for diagnosis and therapy. On an inpatient unit, numerous professionals are involved, including teachers, nurses, occupational and recreational therapists and psychologists in addition to the social worker and psychiatrist. When the pathology includes religious delusions it would seem useful at times to call upon an empathic yet enlightened religious figure from the patient's faith. Such an approach to treatment is not unheard of, as several of the articles compiled by Pattison[45] demonstrate. A religious consultant could help the team members develop a more complete appreciation of the patient's native culture and thereby assist them in becoming more empathic. Of even more importance, this conjoint effort of the team, the consultant, the parents and the child could foster an alliance and result in a more successful psychiatric intervention.

ACKNOWLEDGEMENTS

The authors wish to thank Linda A. Wirth, M.S.S.W. for her assistance; Marc H. Hollender, M.D. and Howard B. Roback, Ph.D. for reviewing the manuscript; and Susan D. Kelton for her help in preparing the manuscript.

REFERENCES

1. Freedman AM, Kaplan HI and Sadock BJ: Comprehensive Textbook of Psychiatry—II. Baltimore, Williams & Wilkins, 1975, p. 2577
2. Wiero, J: De Praestigiis Daemonum et Incantationibus ac Veneficiis. Basel, Oporinus, 1563
3. Mora G: On the 400th anniversary of Johann Weyer's "De Praestigiis Daemonum"—Its significance for today's psychiatry. Am J Psychiatry 120:417–428, 1963
4. Meerloo, JAM: Four hundred years of "witchcraft," "projection" and "delusion." Am J Psychiatry 120:83–6, 1963
5. Lehrman NS: De Praestigiis Daemonum. Am J Psychiatry 120: 1135–6, 1964
6. Freud S: A Seventeenth century demonological neurosis. In: The Complete Psychological Works of Sigmund Freud. Edited by Strachey J. London, Hogarth Press, 1961, pp. 67–105
7. Yap PM: The possession syndrome: a comparison of Hong Kong and French findings. J Ment Sci 106:114–37, 1960
8. Ludwig AM: Witchcraft today. Dis Nerv Sys 26:288–91, 1965
9. Galvin JAV and Ludwig AM: A case of witchcraft. J Nerv Ment Dis 133:161–8, 1961
10. Leininger M: Witchcraft practices and psychocultural therapy with urban US families. Human Organization 32:73–83, 1973
11. Editorial: Exorcism. JAMA 227:1047–8, 1974
12. Greenson RR: Exorcism. JAMA 228:828, 1974
13. Challman A: Exorcism. JAMA 229:140, 1974
14. Bozzuto JC: Cinematic neurosis following "The Exorcist." Report of four cases. J Nerv Ment Dis 161:43–48, 1975
15. Kiraly SJ: Folie à deux. A case of "demonic possession" involving mother and daughter. Can Psychiatr Assoc J 20:223–7, 1975
16. Henderson DJ: Exorcism, possession and the Dracula cult. Bull Menninger Clin 40:603–28, 1976
17. Spiegel D and Fink R: Hysterical psychosis and hypnotizability. Am J Psychiatry 136:777–81, 1979
18. McAll RK: Demonosis or the possession syndrome. Int J Soc Psychiatry 17:150–8, 1971
19. MacKarness R: Occultism and psychiatry. Practitioner 212: 363–6, 1974

20. Casper EG and Philippus MJ: Fifteen cases of embrujada: combining medication and suggestion in treatment. Hosp Community Psychiatry 26:271–4, 1975
21. Cappannari SC, Rau B, Abram HS, et al: Voodoo in the general hospital. A case of hexing and regional enteritis. JAMA 232: 938–40, 1975
22. Lister J: By the London post. N Engl J Med 292:1392–3, 1975
23. Anderson RD: The history of witchcraft: a review with some psychiatric comments. Am J Psychiatry 126:1727–35, 1970
24. Berwick PR and Douglas RR: Hypnosis, exorcism and healing. A case report. Am J Clin Hypn 20:146–8, 1977
25. Bron B: (The phenomenon of possession. Conception and experiences of possession in youth) (German). Confinia Psychiatrica 18:16–29, 1975
26. Cooper PH: The presence of evil in men and places. Practitioner 212:367–9, 1974
27. Cupitt D: Comment. J Med Ethics 2:134–7, 1976
28. Ehrenwald J: Possession and exorcism: delusion shared and compounded. J Am Acad Psychoanal 3:105–9, 1975
29. Figge HH: Spirit possession and healing cult among the Brasilian Umbanda. Psychother Psychosom 25:246–50, 1975
30. Giel R, Gezahegn Y and Luiijk JN van: Faith-healing and spirit-possession in Ghion, Ethiopia. Soc Sci Med 2:63–79, 1968
31. Israel L and North E: (Medicolegal incidence of a delusion of witchcraft: exorcism bringing about the death of a child) (French). Cahiers de Psychiatrie; Supplement au Strasbourg Medical 15:72–85, 1961
32. Nobile C: (On psychoses induced by "witchcraft") (Italian). Cervello 39:277–303, 1963
33. Obeyesekere G: The idiom of demonic possession. A case study. Soc Sci Med 4:97–111, 1970
34. Prince R: Trance and Possession State. Montreal, RM Bucke Memorial Society, 1968
35. Prince WF: Two cures of "paranoia" by experimental appeals to purported obsessing spirits. Psychoanal Rev 56:57–86, 1969
36. Risso M and Böker W: (The delusion of bewitchment. A contribution to the understanding of delusional disorder among the South-Italian workers in Switzerland) (German). Bibliotheca Psychiatrica et Neurologica 124:1–82, 1964
37. Sargant W: The Mind Possessed. Philadelphia, JB Lippincott, 1974
38. Snell JE: Hypnosis in the treatment of the "hexed" patient. Am J Psychiatry 124:311–6, 1967
39. Teoh CL and Dass D: Spirit possession in an Indian family—a case report. Singapore Med J 14:62–4, 1973
40. Trethowan WH: Exorcism: a psychiatric viewpoint. J Med Ethics 2:127–34, 1976
41. Wittkower ED: Trance and possession states. Int J Soc Psychiatry 16:153–60, 1970
42. Wolf MS: Witchcraft and mass hysteria in terms of current psychological theories. J Psychiatr Nurs 14:23–8, 1976
43. Woon TH and Teoh CL: Psychotherapeutic management of a potential spirit medium. Aust N Z J Psychiatry 10:125–8, 1976

44. Pulver SE and Brunt MY: Deflection of hostility in folie à deux. Arch Gen Psychiatry 5:257–65, 1961
45. Pattison EM (editor): Clinical Psychiatry and Religion. Boston, Little Brown & Co., 1969

14

The Possession Syndrome on Trial

RALPH B. ALLISON, *M.D.*[1]

The concept of possession by disincarnate spirits as a cause of mental illness is as old as mankind itself. This belief is still extant in regions of the world where European and American psychiatric belief systems have not replaced older, ritualistic patterns of belief. Scientifically trained observers have reported such cases in the modern literature from exotic locations such as India (1), Egypt (2), New Guinea (3) and Ceylon (4). The most common explanation for such observations is that "spirit possession is a culturally sanctioned, heavily institutionalized and symbolically invested means of expression in action for various ego-dystonic impulses and thoughts." (5)

Closer to home, similar cases of apparent possession have been reported in Latin American countries, such as Columbia. (6) Cases occurring in the United States (7) may be given the Greek label of "caco-demonomania," that is having the delusion of being possessed by demons. (8) The cases described by Schendel and Kourany (8) were of families involved in the charismatic branches of both the Protestant and Catholic religions, leaders of which believe that spirit possession is a major cause of all physical and mental diseases.

In the last decade there has been a resurgence of interest in the emo-

[1]California Mens Colony, San Luis Obispo, California.

Reprinted with permission from *American Journal of Forensic Psychiatry*, 1985, vol. 6, no. 1, 46–56.

tional disorders characterized by the mental mechanism of dissociation, causative of such bewildering conditions as fugue states and multiple personality disorder (MPD). This area of mental illness has a long and controversial history (9), as it deals with that part of the mind which is both fascinating and terrifying to both the sufferer and observer. Therapists treating patients with clearly psychologically created entities, called alter-personalities, may also find themselves confronted with entities for which no internal cause can be discerned and which claim to be entities from outside the patient's mind. (10) Thus, a differential diagnosis becomes necessary for practical reasons, as an alter-personality must be dealt with psychotherapeutically, and an invading spirit must be dealt with by spiritual means.

While dealing with patients who evidence both psychological dissociation and control by invading entities, the therapist becomes quite willing to accept the possibility that "real" possession can exist in vulnerable individuals, and MPD patients are extremely vulnerable, with hatred of their abusing relatives being one of the strongest magnets attracting the "evil entities" into their minds.

The next step in differential diagnosis is between "real" possession and pseudo-possession. The latter condition is better called an "Atypical Dissociative Disorder" (the Possession Syndrome), DSM-III 300.15. (11). A working definition of the Possession Syndrome would be "a dissociative disorder in which the patient unconsciously believes he is possessed by evil spirits who act out his forbidden wishes. The manifestation depends upon his view of what demonic spirits are like and how they should act." Thus, the clinical picture from one individual to another would have little in common, as each person's opinion of what possession is like would be very unique. This is still a mentally created disorder, but different in some of the dynamics from MPD and the other identified dissociative disorders in DSM-III.

The problems in dealing with such a condition in clinical practice are massive enough, but when such a case arises in a forensic setting, the problems multiply. Than at least another differential diagnosis arises, that of playacting or malingering to avoid legal penalties. In addition, the belief systems of the members of the court system must be considered, as they are the ones to make the decisions after hearing the testimony of the witnesses. Such is the case presented below. The details of the case are real; only the names of the persons involved have been fictionalized.

THE CASE OF LEROY JACKSON

On April 11, 1981, police answered a domestic disturbance call from a motel. Upon their arrival, they encountered a short black man named Leroy Jackson who had been having an argument with his wife, Candy, in the presence of her four children by a prior marriage. No one complained of injuries, so the officers did not enter the motel room. Leroy promised to leave, so the police departed.

The motel manager called police again an hour later and they arrested Leroy when they found his 10-year-old stepdaughter, Darnell Thomas, dead of multiple wounds sustained in a beating. Leroy started to run from the police but then turned and surrendered.

The victim had been beaten with a board and with fists during a 22-hour period. She had been choked with a dog chain, put in the attic in a duffle bag and twice had her head rammed into the wall.

Leroy was charged with first degree murder with special circumstances and came to trial in early March of 1982. Just as there appeared to be no possible legal defense and the gas chamber loomed in the distance, his attorney heard testimony from Leroy's wife, Candy, that gave him hope. She testified that, for years, Leroy had spent many long hours talking to himself while alone in a field. He had also called himself "Michael, the Archangel," who had come to rescue this family from the urban ghetto. As Michael, he was most upset that they did not appreciate the sacrifices he had made for them.

Candy also testified that Leroy had frequently called himself "Othello," claiming to be an ex-POW from Greece. As Othello, he forced the children to eat dog food and to drink their own urine.

The attorney called me when he felt he had heard enough to interject an insanity plea in the middle of the ongoing trial. Prior to my arrival, he contracted with a local forensic psychologist to examine Leroy, which he did the day before I came to town. I met with the psychologist and the attorney. The psychologist reported that Leroy could well have MPD, as he had met "Othello Mulett Metheen," a possible alter-personality during the interview. While Leroy consistently claimed amnesia for the day of the crime plus the six days following, Othello readily admitted to having done the killing. I conducted my first interview with Leroy that evening, gathering all the history of dissociative episodes he could recall.

The following day, Saturday, March 13, 1982, the attorney and I conducted a videotaped interview with Leroy in the attorney's office for the purpose of being able to safely present evidence of Leroy's mental state to the court. The taping before noon was a recap of what Leroy had told me the night before, focusing on the several episodes prior to his arrest for which he claimed amnesia. These included three suicide attempts and a tonsillectomy. I then asked him to prepare to let out Othello after lunch, and he agreed, having been aware of Othello for years by virtue of his long conversations with him in the fields. Leroy insisted on being handcuffed behind his back, for our safety. Two deputies were also stationed at the door and window to prevent his escape from the office.

The afternoon taping was of Othello, who managed to twist his handcuffs under his buttocks and get his hands in front of him, where he banged the metal cuffs on the attorney's expensive table, trying to get them off. In a blustering, bragging fashion, he told of killing Darnell, though he would have preferred to have done in her mother, Candy, instead. He showed no remorse and indicated that Leroy had nothing to do with the crime, but he would kill him at a later date.

After Othello's confession, I asked to talk to Michael, the Archangel, but this was unsuccessful. When I tried the procedure used to persuade multiples to switch to a non-dangerous personality, I only succeeded in getting Leroy back. We then showed the videotape to Leroy, as he claimed complete amnesia for that part of the session.

The following Monday I testified that I could make only a provisional diagnosis of the MPD in this case, but I did consider him to be legally insane under current California law. I was unwilling to be definite in my diagnosis until I knew the origin of Othello. I felt that I needed to come back later for another series of interviews when I could pursue the questions that had been raised so far.

During the following month, both sides called in their best forensic psychiatrists and psychologists, nine in all. When I returned five weeks later I was able to read all the reports and discovered that there was a split verdict. Four experts said that the defendant was a multiple; four said he was mentally ill but not a multiple; one said he was faking the whole thing. I was to be the last psychiatrist to testify for the defense prior to submission of the case to the jury

This trip I spent most of Saturday and Sunday (April 17–18, 1982) interviewing Leroy in the county jail. After meeting Leroy briefly I asked to talk to Othello, whom he promptly produced, as he had been produced for any examiner who had asked to talk to him. For the first time, Othello mentioned his son, Joe, so I asked to talk to him. When I met Joe I found an entity who claimed to be the same age as Leroy. He reported being the "snitch" who had told many of the previous examiners what had happened, while they thought they were talking to Leroy. He was willing to tell all about the events relating to the crimes, as well as Leroy's prior experiences, as he had been the former assistant to Othello in doing his evil deeds.

Joe claimed to be a spirit who had last had his own body as a boy in Aukland, New Zealand. He stated that he had fallen off a cliff at the age of 14 and died. He identified Othello as being Lucifer's agent and the one who had accepted the contract from the Council of 12 Arch-demons to kill Leroy's wife, Candy. According to the Council, Candy had been backsliding in her participation in satanic worship services. After breakfast on the day of the crime, Othello took over the body from Leroy and began to threaten Candy by attacking her daughter. His message was, "Agree to be executed, or I'll kill Darnell. I'm knuckling under for nobody." His last threatening act toward Darnell was putting her in a duffle bag and then carrying her to the attic. When that failed to bring Candy around, Othello felt he had to kill somebody to fulfill the contract, so he bashed Darnell's head into the wall, finally killing her.

When Darnell was pulled out of the attic, Joe lost awareness of what was happening. The next thing he remembered was hearing Othello's urgent instructions to run from the police, who had arrived for the second time. As he sprinted away, he looked over his shoulder and saw the glint of gunmetal in the officers' hands. Deciding he wanted to stay alive, he turned and surrendered and was then told that Darnell had died. Prior to that time, he thought she was still alive.

Joe kept control of the body through the booking and initial questioning but relinquished it to Othello the following day. Othello held sway from the next six days, when Leroy came to being beaten by other inmates when they discovered he was a "baby killer."

Joe explained the first appearance of Othello to Leroy, at age four. Leroy's divorced mother worked all day and left her children in the care of Jack, her brutal boyfriend. Jack locked Leroy in a closet while he sexually molested Leroy's sisters. Finally, neighbors called police, who removed the children from the home, but they missed Leroy in the closet. His mother came home to find her children gone, a note from the police on the kitchen table and Leroy still hiding in the closet under the clothes hems. As Joe said, "A person feels like he has been mistreated and thrown around, sexually assaulted. This builds up and makes a four-year-old turn away. They said there is a God. How come you don't do something? He doesn't understand. Here's a male doll in a dark closet. Used it for a type of voodoo. He took it, talked to it as a friend and wished. He talked to the doll. Why was Jack doing what he was doing? How could he get back? He felt lonely, not many playmates. Othello came in from the outside and gave orders. Son of fire, water and ice."

Joe explained that archdemons are strongest on Wednesdays and Saturdays. (The killing took place on a Saturday.) That is why I came to see him on a Sunday, which was the strongest day of the week for Michael, the Archangel. This time when I asked to talk to Michael, I was successful, in spite of interference from Othello.

Here are his words: "I am Michael. I am a warrior. I've been with him five years now."

I asked why.

"For a young man who was born possessed with the evilness of Lucifer, for the life that was cast away, like the fire that burns away. Now the child is grown and the days are shorter. For then Othello exists. The battle continues till lives are taken. No more blood shall be stricken from the earth."

I asked, "Why didn't you prevent the murder?"

"You have twelve demons who exist. I don't win every battle that exists."

I asked, "Did Leroy make you?"

"He didn't make me."

I asked, "Where are you?"

"Like an angel, as in the Bible, I am in that rank."

The next day in court, Leroy was in legal chains and handcuffs since Othello was determined to come out and give a statement, invited or not. He did take over the body, as manifested with intense shuffling and muttering, in contrast to Leroy's usual quiet and passive behavior. In my testimony I concluded that Leroy Jackson did not fit the MPD but rather the Possession Syndrome, an Atypical Dissociative Disorder. My theory was that what we had observed was a creation of Leroy's unconscious mind and was simply a dramatic picture of what he wished to be and do but could not see as himself.

Following my testimony, the jury found him guilty of first degree murder with special circumstances. During the penalty phase, Othello was allowed to testify. He told the all white "honky jury" that he didn't care what they said since Leroy was going to die by his, Othello's, hand that December on his twin son's birthday. Then he, Othello, would move on to another living body.

The jury found him sane and sentenced him to death.

DISCUSSION

In working out my final diagnostic formulation, I felt that there were four major differential diagnoses to consider in this case: malingering, MPD, "real" possession and the Possession Syndrome. None of these is easy to diagnose in and of itself, and differentiating them is even harder. The scientific literature offers the psychiatrist only scant guidelines. Varma, Bouri and Wig (12) noted only two out of five characteristics to distinguish their case of multiple personality from the "Hysterical Possession Syndrome" in their Indian cases. The hysterically possessed subject is aware of the abnormal personality while the multiple is not, and the entity is a deity, spirit or known person in the hysterically possessed patient, while the alter-personality is no known person and is the manifestation of conflict in the multiple. But I had to come to some logical conclusion from the data so far collected.

Since there was data presented by witnesses that he had shown at least Othello and Michael on numerous occasions prior to the arrest, those entities had not been fabricated to provide him with a defense. There was also hard evidence, including police and hospital reports, to verify Joe's stories about conduct during Leroy's amnesic periods. Despite the efforts of the District Attorney to portray this odd behavior as nothing more than the play acting of an unsophisticated ghetto youth who was attempting to fool the experts, the evidence was there to show that the manifestations of this illness had existed for at least a decade.

Several factors weighed against my picking MPD as the most likely diagnosis,—the subject's choice of victim was one important item. He had many times in the past indicated his fondness for the victim, to the point where her mother had become jealous of his attentions to Darnell. The defendant had tried his best to be the father none of these children had, in his persona of Leroy Jackson, and he really had no motive to kill this child, as she had not done anything to anger him so.

There was, however, ample reason for him to hate Candy, but more than likely he repressed those urges, in order to continue to see himself as the devoted husband. Candy had a long documented history of beating all of her children. She had been threatened with arrest for this behavior in several states. Joe reported that most of the beating by hand that Darnell received immediately prior to her death was delivered by her mother, not by Leroy. Candy was Leroy's woman, and he was too nice a guy to hate her, as far as he was consciously aware. What lurked in his unconscious mind was another story. In my experience with bona fide MPD patients who did kill, the victim was a person the patient had personally hated and perceived as his persecutor. He did not displace his anger onto an innocent victim.

Another important difference was the reported nature of the origin of the hostile entity, Othello. The description usually given by a multiple of the origin of the first hostile alter-personality usually relates to an attack by some adult he had trusted for care, a parent, for example. In this case the villain was Jack, mother's boyfriend. Jack was not described as one Leroy could or should trust, as he was assigned to care for all the children while Mother worked. I could perceive no positive affection on Leroy's part for Jack nor any expectation of his liking Jack at all. His total affect for Jack was, in fact, hatred. This hatred was then displaced onto a demon he made and named Othello, who could carry it for him. When a potential multiple is overwhelmingly abused by a parent he should love, he splits a part of himself off to become a nonpersonal entity who can then hate the parent of that other person who still loves the abusing adult. Leroy did not deny Othello's existence and carried on many long conversations with him over the years. This is something the multiple would not be expected to do, as he must deny this evil intent toward someone he believes he is expected to love. The multiple is unaware of the hostile entity he has created. Leroy was good friends with his own.

Leroy used the mental mechanism of identification with the aggressor to design Othello, using Jack as his model. The types of abuse he described which Jack imposed on him and his sisters were exactly the same as Candy described Othello imposing on her children, namely eating dog food, drinking urine and being tied up with dog chains. While the same mechanism of defense may be used by a multiple in a later alter-personality creation, it is not likely to be used the first time. At that time, he is more likely to create an entity whom the abusing parent will like, one that can survive despite the abuse heaped upon him. This will most likely be a compliant entity rather than an angry and hostile one and is thus likely to invite more wrath from someone like Jack.

Differentiating from "real" possession is even more difficult, since one has to assume that such a condition does exist. If it does, then it should follow rules which are common to all religions. In Leroy's case, there was a major flaw in the repeated insistence that God is strongest on Sundays and on Wednesdays and Saturdays the Archdemons are strongest. The Gregorian calendar was, after all, man-made, and I personally know of no religion that proclaims that God does more work on one day of the week than on another. Leroy's concept did not seem to me to be theologically sound.

Another flaw was that Othello was so easy to reach and so ready to come out to have his say. If he really was an evil spirit, he had no need to restrict himself to Leroy's body and could have done all he wanted to upset the trial by non-physical means. I saw no rationale for an evil spirit emerging so baldly and identifying itself. It would seem to me more logical for him to do his dirty deeds without such advertisement of his existence.

There was also evidence that Othello had engaged in pimping prostitutes, selling drugs, stealing explosives from National Guard armories and engaging in other unlawful activities, all of which were unknown to Leroy. All of these activities seemed more appropriate for an entity that expressed Leroy's hatred of the society he lived in rather than a demon spirit doing the work of Satan.

POSTSCRIPT

Two years after his conviction, on July 20, 1984, I conducted a four-hour interview with Leroy in a locked contact booth in the prison's visiting area. Leroy arrived, appearing cheerful, sporting a mustache and reading glasses. The interview lasted four hours. During this time I also reviewed matters with Othello and Joe, both of whom appeared with the cooperation of Leroy. No one knew what had happened to Archangel Michael, and he did not make an appearance at that time. Overall, there seemed to be no change in the balance of forces I had observed during the trial, since three of the entities were still in attendance and had been active during the previous years of incarceration.

Leroy was very proud to report that he had learned to read, write and type in prison. His main accomplishment had been to secure official records through his sister, which proved to him that the District Attorney was completely wrong in asserting that he had lied about the incidents of child abuse in his past. Now that he could read the court testimony documents, he knew what facts he needed to prove to show he had been truthful in his statements to the psychiatrists, and he had secured court and police documents that verified his own memory. He had done this, not for the purpose of going back and re-trying his case but to be absolutely sure of his own roots and confident of his own recollections. Being called a liar by the District Attorney was something he could not let go unchallenged.

The patient is getting along well with all staff and the civilized inmates, but some of the inmates do know him as Othello. He stays in his cell most of the time since he cannot risk letting Othello out among other inmates. He is still communicating with Othello regularly, but, as he says, "on my own terms." Leroy is still experiencing amnesic episodes. Othello did not execute him on his son's birthday in December, 1982, as threatened in court, however Leroy did awaken in his cell with multiple bleeding slash wounds of his right forearm on January 13, 1984 and required hospitalization. Leroy believes that Othello is trying to tear away at his body, bit by bit. He exhibited to me the 20 gash wound scars on his right inner forearm.

Leroy made no requests for me to intervene in any way in his situation. He reiterated orally what he had earlier written to me: "I still have this problem and all I want is to die; then I won't have to live like this."

When I asked Leroy to let me talk to Othello, he reluctantly agreed but stalled as long as he could. Finally, his face became expressionless with his eyes wide open for a minute. Then, the voice I knew to be Othello's came forth, with its usual gutter language, in contrast to Leroy's polite English.

Othello did not recognize me, since he had expected someone else, so I introduced myself to him. He referred to himself as the "King" and indicated a distinct pleasure in being in a prison where there were so many of his old gang buddies from the ghetto. He was apparently up to all of the old illegal tricks that he played outside prison and behaved like any convict who did all he could to defy the authorities while in prison. He told me that Candy was in prison, while Leroy had no idea where she was now.

It was apparent to me, now that Othello was out, that he would prefer to stay out, but that was not to my liking. I did not dare let him out into the visiting area where he could easily ruin Leroy's good reputation with the correctional officers. Also, I was locked into this steel and plexiglass booth and had no way to leave if Othello should get angry with me. I asked him to let Joe come out for his turn, but he was not eager to give way to that traitor, and I had to devise a strategy to get him to leave on his own accord when I was done with him. Besides two chairs, the only items in the booth were an ashtray and a Bible. I picked up the Bible and leafed through it to get his attention. Then I casually brushed it against his left elbow. With that touch, he became testy but not hostile. He objected to my gesture but I also sensed that he feared it. Not long after my move, he quieted down, his face went blank and, with his eyes still open, he left, to be replaced by Joe, his former assistant assassin.

With a sigh of relief, I held a long conversation with Joe about current events. His job is to protect the body from harm and to do all he can to get a better deal for Leroy. Although he has no hope that Leroy can be cured of his "cancer" of 28 years, he is the entity who meets with the defense attorneys to develop legal strategies for further hearings on Leroy's case.

In Joe's opinion, if Leroy is executed by the State, Othello will simply go back to being a soul again and will join with someone else to continue his evil deeds. The next time it will take someone stronger than Michael to stop him from killing again. He asked to go when he had said enough and to let Leroy return.

When Leroy awoke he wondered why he had not been wearing his glasses. (Neither Othello nor Joe needs glasses.) I briefly informed him of what had transpired, which did not seem to surprise him. A friendly correctional officer came by and, like friendly associates, they gleefully waved to each other. After locating an officer who would unlock the door, I said farewell and returned to the outside world.

CONCLUSIONS

Two years on Death Row has apparently not changed the essential psychodynamic picture of Leroy Jackson. Now in prison, while the angelic rescuer has disappeared from view, Leroy, Othello and Joe have split up the required roles of any long-term prison inmate. Leroy deals with the staff and the relatively civilized inmates, makes friends, follows the rules and is duly respected for his proper institutional behavior. He conducts research into his own personal past for the purpose of proving his memory correct and for disproving the prosecution's accusations that he lied in court.

Othello, the antisocial entity, is playing life in prison by the inmate code; he will do anything he can and get away with. He associates with the same people he did when he was in the ghetto and behaves in the same way as when he lived there.

Joe, the advocate and rescuer, is working with the attorneys to obtain an appeal hearing and secure a legal basis for overturning the death sentence. In the meantime, he is doing what he can to keep Leroy safe from Othello's attempts to harm or kill the body they share.

Such is the current state of affairs with this little band of entities that share Leroy Jackson's body and consciousness. I see no reason to alter my trial testimony; the psychological processes then described still go on, regardless of what those around him may believe. Those who work with Leroy Jackson in the areas mentioned will need all the skill, enlightenment and ingenuity they can assemble for the task.

REFERENCES

1. Teja JS, Khanna BA, Subrahmanyam, TB: "Possession states" in Indian patients. Indian J Psychiatry 12:71–87, 1970
2. Nelson, C: Spirit possession and world view: an illustration from Egypt. Int J Soc Psychiatry 17:194–209, 1971
3. Salisbury RF: Possession in the New Guinea highlands. Int J Soc Psychiatry 14:85–94, 1968
4. Obeysekere G: The idiom of demonic possession: a case study. Soc Sci & Med 4:97–111, 1970
5. Kiev A: Spirit possession in Haiti. Am J Psychiatry 118:133, 1961, Quoted by Teja (1970)
6. Leon CA: "El duende" and other incubi: suggestive interactions between culture, the devil, and the brain. Arch Gen Psychiatry 32:155–162, 1975
7. Ludwig AM: Witchcraft today. Dis Nerv Syst 26:288–291, 1965
8. Schendel E & Kourany RC: Cacodemonomania and exorcism in children. J Clin Psychiatry 41:119–123, 1980
9. Ellenberger HF. The Discovery of the Unconscious. The History and Evolution of Dynamic Psychiatry. New York: Jason Aronson, 1976
10. Allison RB & Schwartz T: Minds in Pieces. New York: Rawson Wade, 1980

11. Diagnostic and Statistical Manual of Mental Disorders, Third Edition, Washington, DC: APA, 1980
12. Varma VK, Bouri M, Wig NN: Multiple personality in India: comparison with hysterical possession state. Am J Psychother 25:113–120, 1981

15

Cacodemonomania

PAULA H. SALMONS,
MB, CHB, MRC PSYCH,[1]
DAVID J. CLARKE

"There is also, concerning witches who copulate with devils, much difficulty in considering the methods by which such abominations are consummated. . . . the Inquisitor of Como in the County of Burbia, who in the space of one year, which was the year of grace 1485, caused forty-one witches to be burned; who all publicly affirmed, as it is said, that they had practised these abominations with devils."

Malleus Maleficarum. (1486).

The experience of having had intercourse with the devil has in the past been regarded as evidence that the individual is a witch. Those investigating cases of witchcraft were advised to seek the judgment of doctors, and the verdict of physicians became a test for the presence or absence of witchcraft. The woman described in this case study might well have suffered the death penalty in former times. She is unusual because of her belief that she had had intercourse with the Devil, and because the belief was shared by her religious minister. The patient also presents a diagnostic problem.

[1]University of Birmingham, England.

Reprinted with permission from *Psychiatry*, 1987, vol. 50, 50–54. Copyright 1987 by William Alanson White Psychiatric Foundation.

A 38-year-old, married, woman teacher, Mrs. A, was admitted from Out-Patients in 1984 with a history of feelings of unreality, alterations in mood and expressions of the belief that she was possessed by an evil god that made her carry out actions against her will. Two years previously, while she was reading the New Testament, a "force" inside her suggested that she could have more pleasurable sensations than those to be obtained while reading the Bible. She lay down on the bed and had sexual intercourse with the force, "as with a man," and with the physical sensation of penetration, resulting in orgasm. Since then there had been about 12 similar instances—some pleasurable but most not. She said it had not been pleasurable recently and described it as "filthy." Her sexual relationship with her husband had declined, and she now felt that intercourse was repulsive.

Mrs. A's history had started 5 years previously, in 1979, when she had presented feeling low in mood, lethargic and detached from events occurring around her. A diagnosis of depersonalization syndrome with atypical depression was made. Treatment with dexamphetamine produced elevation of mood but accompanied by overconfidence and aggression. After a traffic accident, her treatment was changed to methylphenidate.

Over the next 2 years the feelings of unreality and depression persisted, and treatment with tranylcypromine was started. Shortly afterward, while lying in bed, the patient became convinced that her husband had physically altered. He felt scaly to the touch, and when she looked at him, she saw several extra eyes and limbs. The episode passed after some minutes but was followed by marked mood swings lasting a few days at a time, with periods of elation and overactivity alternating with lowered mood and anergia.

One day while sitting in the bath, Mrs. A became convinced that she was shedding large pieces of skin, which she could see and which were blocking the drain hole. Shortly afterward all drugs were stopped because the patient had become pregnant with her third child. There were no complications during pregnancy and labor, and a normal female infant was delivered.

Mrs. A's psychiatric condition remained unchanged until the child was 4 months old. While sitting at home, she suddenly smelled an overpowering odor, "just like a newborn baby," although her daughter was in a different room. Later she suddenly had the conviction that her daughter's skin was peeling off and that some of the skin was wrapped around the refrigerator in the kitchen.

Until this time, Mrs. A's religious beliefs, which were of an orthodox Christian nature, had not changed. However, a few months later, in 1982, while attending a Bible class, she began to feel that her god was different in some way from the god that other people experienced. She said, "The word Jesus is now anathema to me." She had been forced by her god to tear up the New Testament section of her Bible, which she put in a brown paper bag and posted through her religious minister's door.

Mrs. A had a miscarriage in 1983 (her fourth pregnancy), and a few months later she suddenly knew that the baby would be presented to her by her god if she searched for it in some nearby woods. She rushed from the house in night attire and bare feet, ripping her clothes and cutting herself in her struggle through the woods.

Mrs. A often had "funny turns," in which she would feel unwell and have a sense of unreality. In three of these she was made to turn the gas taps of her cooker on "by the god in possession in me," and in another, the sleeve of her pullover caught fire while she was cooking and burned her skin.

When admitted in 1984, Mrs. A gave the additional history that over the previous 6 months the god that possessed her had had intercourse with her several times. She also described how one evening she became convinced that her own face had changed, the left side below her eye becoming horny and detached from the rest of her face.

PATIENT'S PERSONAL HISTORY

Mrs. A had been adopted at the age of 3 months, and no information was available about her natural parents. Her adoptive parents were both alive and well; her father had been a factory worker.

Early infancy and childhood had been unremarkable. She left school after passing her public examinations in two subjects, later taking a correspondence course which led to certificates in a further five subjects. She worked as a junior school (5-year-olds) teacher for a while before going to teachers' training college. Subsequently she taught physical training in a secondary school until she left at the age of 28 to start a family.

The patient had married at 23. Her husband, who was 4 years older, was a teacher, a quiet man who had little contact with people outside the family. The marriage appeared stable. At the time of hospital admission, the couple's three girls were aged 10, 7 and 3 years. Mr. A appeared unconcerned about all the peculiar happenings and continued to go to work regularly.

Mrs. A presented as neatly and well dressed. Her appearance and behavior were appropriate, and superficially she established reasonable rapport. Her speech and language were normal, although she was evasive when asked to describe her abnormal experiences; it was difficult to clarify her emotions and experiences. Her affect was always appropriate but emotionally "cool." There was no evidence of thought disorder, and cognitive function was intact.

Physical examination and routine investigations were entirely normal. EEGs carried out at the start of her illness indicated that during overbreathing, bitemporal 7 Hertz rhythmic activity occurred. Subsequently, the EEG was completely normal. A 48-hour EEG showed that during sleep stages one and two, occasional beta activity was seen in the left posterior temporal derivations. It was not typical of epilepsy. A CT scan of the skull showed some minor symmetrical prominence of both lateral ventricles. This did not alter over the course of the subsequent two years and was not thought to have clinical significance.

The patient declined treatment after her admission examinations, saying that her problems were spiritual, not medical. Her young religious minister agreed that Mrs. A was possessed by a malevolent force, which was responsible for all the events. On several occasions, he claimed, his treatment with prayers had stopped her peculiar feelings—especially her hatred of Jesus. He felt that medical treatment was inappropriate, and he clearly reinforced her beliefs.

DISCUSSION

There is evidence that a belief in witchcraft is still prevalent in modern Western society (see, e.g., Galvin et al. 1962). Edwards and Gill (1981) have drawn attention to three recent cases reported in the press in which tragedies occurred as the result of attempts at exorcism. They suggest that the popularity of the occult as a subject for plays, films and books is evidence of widespread lay interest, and they contrast this with the lack of recent discussion in medical and psychiatric journals.

In the French literature earlier this century, Vinchon (1931) had distinguished three types of possession: hysteria, anxiety nightmares and those due to a dissociative process. Several French authors described different types of cases and possession (Schiff and Simon 1933; Delay 1945; Mars 1946). Lhermitte (1944) published extensively and is regarded as an authority. However, he viewed possession states from the position of an orthodox Catholic psychiatrist and accepted the cooperation of the exorcist. He distinguished "true" possession from "false" possession, identifying the former as instances where a psychiatric explanation was not adequate or plausible. These views appear to be shared by more recent clerical writers. Henry Cooper (1974), Rector of St. George's Church, Bloomsbury, felt that a major difficulty in cases of possession presenting to the clergy was diagnosis. He advised that except in cases of emergency, causes other than true possession by an evil force should be excluded by consultation with the patient's doctors. His conclusion, however, was that "there seems to be a small, and increasing percentage of cases in which the presence of objective evil is the only reasonable conclusion to draw." Cooper advocates the intelligent use of exorcism in cooperation with the medical profession.

In Yap's study of 66 cases in Hong Kong (1960), delusions of possession were most prevalent in divorced women who came from a low socioeconomic background and who were illiterate. His most common diagnosis was hysteria. The patients he described were clearly unsophisticated, and he could identify precipitating causes in 20% of the cases. Only two of his cases had experience of coitus with the possessing spirit. This contrasts with Lucas et al. (1962), who studied over 400 schizophrenic patients. The most common delusion in both sexes was of imposed heterosexual activity; it was most prominent in unmarried females.

More recently, Schendel and Kourany (1980) described cacodemonomania in five children. In at least three of the cases, the belief in demon possession was initiated by someone other than the child. The authors described the clinical situation as a folie à deux syndrome in which one or more members of the family shared the child's delusion. All five children in his study had suffered the loss of a natural parent; in three of these instances the remaining parent had remarried. Raschka (1979) also drew attention to the link between parental deprivation and delusional sexual experiences. This link had first been interpreted by Freud, in his paper, "A Seventeenth-Century Demonological Neurosis." He described the possession of a young man with melancholia who had made a pact with the Devil. Freud interpreted the Devil in this case to be a substitute for the father, whose death had originally precipitated the melancholia. Bozzuto (1975) reinterprets this to mean retention of a part object in the face of loss as a partial solution to that loss. Anderson (1970) extended this idea from the individual to the cultural when he suggested that 15th-century Christianity attempted to resolve oedipal conflicts with the concepts of a good God-father and an evil or sexual Devil-father.

Kenny (1981) discusses the phenomenological similarities between possession states and multiple personality. In both conditions, the individual experiences a period of time in which traits sharply contrasting with the "normal" are exhibited. In either state, possession or multiple personality, normally unacceptable impulses or wishes can be expressed.

Trethowan (1976) points out that delusions of possession can indicate a psychotic illness, in which the notion of being possessed may be symptomatic of the disturbance of ego functioning occurring in schizophrenia—a passivity experience. Severely neurotic patients may exhibit hysterical and other symptoms resembling those occurring in possession states.

Possession states are clearly more prevalent in some cultures than others. A belief in demonology and the occurrence of these syndromes has been thought to be coincident with an oppressive social structure and an inability to cope with its evils (Wijesinghe et al. 1976). It is clear from reports from other cultures that such states may provide a socially sanctioned behavioral outlet for repressed impulses and needs and do not necessarily represent psychiatric illness (Yap 1960; Kiev 1961). What is interesting, though, is that even in a Western culture in which demoniacal belief is not an active part of orthodox religious practice, such syndromes still arise, and similarities occur between patients from widely differing cultures. For instance, in common with patients described elsewhere, Mrs. A had lost both of her natural parents. Although her adoption at an early age provided an apparently adequate environment, she was nevertheless aware of her loss. Her delusional ideas, although not prevalent in her culture, clearly were part of the subculture in which she lived, and they were shared, apparently, by those in her village and certainly by her minister. She refused medical treatment, as did the patients described by Schendel and Kourany and by Leon (1975). However, unlike the patients described by Yap, she was middle class and educated.

The patient described here presented some diagnostic difficulties—the profusion of symptoms was difficult to combine in a single diagnosis. The delusional belief occurred fairly late in the course of the disorder, and was prominent. This leads to the suspicion of a psychotic illness. However, at that time, disturbance of affect was not marked, and there were no biological features of depression. Apart from the delusional ideas and the apparent hallucinatory experiences, there were no other features suggestive of a schizophrenic disorder.

The multiplicity of symptoms, including depersonalization phenomena and alterations in level of consciousness, could be accounted for by a hysterical neurosis. The patient was probably receiving some secondary gain from the attention of her minister and her notoriety in the village where she lived. Since her minister shared her beliefs, one could postulate a folie à deux syndrome in which Mrs. A was the principal (Dewhurst and Todd 1956) although she was not psychotic.

In view of the olfactory, tactile and visual hallucinations reported, other diagnoses, such as temporal lobe epilepsy, have been considered, but the evidence for this from EEG studies is lacking.

The discussion that took place with the patient's minister illustrates a problem occasionally encountered in psychiatric practice. The psychiatrist's belief system (that the patient's symptoms represented psychiatric disorder) had no common ground with the patient's belief system or her minister's. Her minister asserted that he had read the world theological literature on possession states and that he had no doubt that Mrs. A had a spiritual and not a psychiatric disorder.

Several psychiatrists investigating these disorders have felt that the efforts of a single discipline are inadequate to deal with such complex spiritual problems (Edward and Gill; Leon; Schendel and Kourany). Edwards and Gill developed a working group comprising two members of the clergy, a psychiatrist with religious convictions and an agnostic psychiatrist, so that a better understanding of the patient's problems could be achieved. Although patients like Mrs. A present only infrequently, psychiatrists should not be waylaid into always viewing them within the narrow confines of psychiatric diagnosis. A broader perspective is required, which takes account not only of the patient's interpersonal difficulties but also of the individual's subculture and spiritual life.

REFERENCES

Anderson, R. D. The history of witchcraft: A review with some psychiatric comments. *American Journal of Psychiatry* (1970) 126:69–77.

Bozzuto, J. C. Cinematic neurosis following *The Exorcist*. *Journal of Nervous and Mental Disease* (1975) 161:43–48.

Cooper, H. C. The Presence of evil in men and places. *The Practitioner* (1974) 212:367–69.

Delay, J. Delire de possession diabolique. *Presse Medicale* (1945) 11:143.

Dewhurst, K., and Todd, J. The psychosis of association—folie à deux. *Journal of Nervous and Mental Disease* (1956) 124:451–59.

Edwards, J. G., and Gill, D. Psychiatry and the occult. *The Practitioner* (1981) 225:83–88.

Freud, S. A seventeenth-century demonological Neurosis (1923). *Standard Edition of the Complete Psychological Works*, Vol. 19. Hogarth, 1961.

Galvin, J. A. V., and Ludwig, A. M. A case of witchcraft. *Journal of Nervous and Mental Disease* (1962) 133:161–68.

Kenny, M. G. Multiple personality and spirit possession. *Psychiatry* (1981) 44:337–58.

Kiev, A. Spirit possession in Haiti. *American Journal of Psychiatry* (1961) 118:133–38.

Léon, C. A. "El Duende" and other incubi. *Archives of General Psychiatry* (1975) 32:155–62.

Lhermitte, J. Les psychoses de possession diabolique. *Revue Medicale Française* (1944) 4:51–54.

Lucas, C.J., Sainsbury, P., and Collins, J. G. A social and clinical study of delusions in schizophrenia. *Journal of Mental Science* (1962) 108:747–58.

Malleus Maleficarum [1486]. London: Arrow Books, 1971.

Mars, L. *La Crise de possession dans le Vaudou*. Port-au-Prince: Imprimerie de l'Etat, 1946.

Raschka, L. B. The incubus syndrome: A variant of erotomania. *Canadian Journal of Psychiatry* (1979) 24:549–53.

Schendel, E., and Kourany, R. F. C. Cacodemonomania and exorcism in children. *Journal of Clinical Psychiatry* (1980) 41(4):119–23.

Schiff, P., and Simon, R. Delire de possession zoopathique succedant à un delire de gross sesse chez un obese post-encephalitique. *Annales Medico-Psychologiques* (1933) 91:612–15.

Trethowan, W. H. Exorcism: A psychiatric viewpoint. *Journal of Medical Ethics* (1976) 2:127–34.

Vinchon, J. In M. Laignel-Lavastine, ed., *The Concentric Method in the Diagnosis of Psychoneurotics*. London: Kegan, Paul, Trench, Trubner, 1931.

Wijesinghe, C. P., Dissanayake, S. A. W., and Mendis, N. (1976). Possession trance in a semiurban community in Sri Lanka. *Australia and New Zealand Journal of Psychiatry* (1976) 10:135–39.

Yap, P. M. The Possession syndrome: A comparison of Hong Kong and French findings. *Journal of Mental Science* (1960) 106:114–37.

Name Index

Subject Index

RICHARD NOLL, PH.D., is a clinical psychologist and a freelance writer. He is in private practice in Philadelphia. He completed an externship at New York University Medical Center in New York City and was formerly a staff clinical psychologist for four years at Ancora Psychiatric Hospital in Hammonton, New Jersey. Dr. Noll recently received his doctorate in clinical psychology at the New School for Social Research in New York. The author of many scholarly articles on psychiatric and anthropological topics, he is also the author of a forthcoming reference work, *The Encyclopedia of Schizophrenia and the Psychotic Disorders*. Dr. Noll has a long-standing interest in unusual psychiatric syndromes and in the history and folklore of psychopathology.

In October 1991 the author completed a lecture tour in Eastern Europe during which he spoke on both psychiatric and anthropological topics. He delivered a presentation to an interdisciplinary organization of Polish scientists and academics at the Royal Castle in Warsaw on the latest scientific research on multiple personality and the dissociative disorders and the relevance of the work of C. G. Jung to this topic. He also lectured on both multiple personality and shamanism at the universities in Warsaw, Kielce, and Kraków, Poland. In addition, Dr. Noll spoke on the psychological aspects of shamanism, and he conducted research on the subject of Central European witchcraft at the Ethnographic Institute of the Hungarian Academy of Sciences in Budapest, Hungary.